MEMORY NOTEBOOK OF NURSING

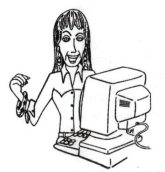

JoAnn Zerwekh, EdD, RN, FNP

Executive Director
Nursing Education Consultants
Dallas, Texas

Nursing Faculty
University of Phoenix
Phoenix, Arizona

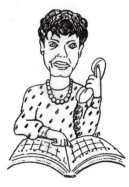

Jo Carol Claborn, MS, RN

Executive Director
Nursing Education Consultants
Dallas, Texas

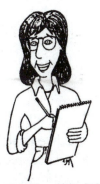

CJ Miller, BSN, RN

Nurse-Illustrator

Nursing Education Consultants
Ingram ★ Texas

Artist: C.J. Miller, RN
Washington, Iowa

Production Manager: Mike Cull
Gingerbread Press, Waxahachie, Texas
Desktop Publishing Assistant: James Halfast
San Angelo, Texas

◆

◆

Printed in the United States of America

Nursing Education Consultants
P O Box 465
Ingram, Texas 78025
(800) 933-7277

ISBN: 1892155125 (9781892155122)

Library of Congress Catalog Number: 2007939690

◆

Any procedure or practice described in this book should be applied by the health-care practitioner under appropriate supervision in accordance with professional standards of care used with regard to the unique circumstances that apply in each practice situation. Care has been taken to confirm the accuracy of information presented and to describe generally accepted practices, however, the authors, editors, and publisher cannot accept any responsibility for errors or omissions or for consequences from application of the information in this book and make no warranty, express or implied, with respect to the contents of this book.

This book is written to be used as a study aid and review book for nursing. It is not intended for use as a primary resource for procedures, treatments, medications or to serve as a complete textbook for nursing care.

Copies of this book may be obtained directly from Nursing Education Consultants. (1-800-846-TEXT).

Last Digit is the Print Number: 5 4 3 2 1

CONTRIBUTORS & REVIEWERS

Joanna Barnes, MSN, RN
ADN Program Coordinator
Grayson College
Denison, Texas

Susan Priest, MSN, RN, CSN
Nursing Faculty
Alvin Community College
Alvin, Texas

Sharon Decker, RN, PhD, CS, CCRN, ANEF
Professor and Director of Clinical Simulations
Texas Tech University Health Sciences Center
School of Nursing
Lubbock, Texas

Sylvia Rayfield, MN, RN
Sylvia Rayfield & Associates
Gulf Shores, Alabama

Catherine Rosser EdD, CNA-BC, RN
Undergraduate Program Director
Louise Herrington School of Nursing
Baylor University
Dallas, Texas

Barbara Devitt, MSN, RN
Nursing Faculty
Louise Herrington School of Nursing
Baylor University
Dallas, Texas

Kim Sherer, MN, RN
Northern Oklahoma College
Tonkawa, Oklahoma

Bobbi Emmons, MS, RN
Northern Oklahoma College
Tonkawa, Oklahoma

Linda Stevenson, PhD, RN
Louise Herrington School of Nursing
Baylor University
Dallas, Texas

Lt Col (Ret) Michael Hutton, MSN, RN
Nursing Faculty
Blinn College
Brady Texas

Mary Ann Yantis, EdD, RN
Louise Herrington School of Nursing
Baylor University
Dallas, Texas

Alice Pappas, PhD, RN
Clinical Research Nurse
Childrens Hospital Boston
Boston, MA

ACKNOWLEDGMENTS

From the authors: We want to express our appreciation to the students of our review courses and readers of our books. The inspiration for this book came from your encouragement and enthusiasm. It is for you, the student, that this book was created.

We thank our children — Ashley Garneau, Tyler Zerwekh, Jaelyn Conway, Michael Brown, and Kimberley Aultman for tolerating our ups and downs as this manuscript was prepared. We especially want to thank Robert Claborn for his continued patience and support of all of our activities. JoAnn wishes to acknowledge John Masog for his warm presence in her life, sense of humor, and willingness to be a part of it all.

From the illustrator: I would like to thank my children Nathan and Kimberly for all of their support and encouragement as well as the many great friends that have come and stayed in my life throughout the years.

Our sincere appreciation to:

James Halfast our graphics production manager, who juggles NEC with his family and work schedule;

Mike Cull and all the support staff at CuLeGo for their persistence and patience in working with us;

Elaine Nokes for keeping our office running smoothly while we're buried in our books;

Dave Meier from the Center for Accelerated Learning at Lake Geneva, Wisconsin for introducing us to these ideas to help students learn;

And to Lucy Claborn who continues to inspire us with her humor, courage and spirit! We love you very much.

Preface

Memory Notebook of Nursing, Vol 1 was the first of the series of the Memory Notebooks of Nursing. We are so pleased that you have enjoyed the images and mnemonics over the years and we are excited to bring you yet another edition. This one, as the last, continues to utilize the unique visual approach to learning. This edition will continue to assist you in studying, reviewing and presenting information. It is a great tool for the nursing student who is struggling through the enormous amount of material in nursing school as well as for the new graduate who is preparing for the National Council Licensure Examination. Nursing Education Consultants has continued to utilize the principles of accelerated learning and humorous visual images to provide an appealing and humorous approach to remembering important information. This approach is made possible by the illustrations of C.J. Miller, who is also a nurse.

First, a little information about accelerated learning and how you can enhance your learning by utilizing both the left (analytical, linear, logical, rote memory) side of your brain and the right (visual, images, musical, imaginative) side of your brain. Several techniques are used to encourage the whole-brain to think and learn concepts. These techniques are memory tools, mindmapping, and mnemonics. Memory tools are aids to assist you to draw associations from other ideas with the use of visual images to help cement the learning. Mindmapping ™ was developed by Tony Buzan as a tool to help people take notes more effectively. Mindmapping is in sharp contrast to the traditional method of taking notes in an outline form. Instead, a thought or concept is written in the center of the page, images and color are added to information as ideas begin to flow out from the center focus. Another technique is the use of mnemonics. Mnemonics are most often words, phrases, or sentences that help you remember information. Throughout this book you will find ideas that we have found useful in teaching students and nurses how to remember information. As you read over each illustration, get involved with the process and write down your own ideas on the drawings. Think about this, color activates the brain and music increases right brain activity. Time to get out the crayolas and color the pictures. As you are coloring or writing, turn on some music, don't be afraid to experiment - find out what type of music works best for you.

If you really like the Memory Notebook of Nursing, Vol 1, then check out our other Memory Notebooks of Nursing. Memory Notebook of Nursing Vol 2, 3rd edition has more great images and mnemonics, Memory Notebook of Nursing: Pharmacology and Diagnostics provides a great study tool for Pharmacology. Same great concepts – but different images and mnemonics. Check out the inside of the back cover of this book for more information

The authors of this book also have NCLEX Examination review books for both PN's and RN's – Illustrated Study Guide for the NCLEX RN Examination, and Illustrated Study Guide for the NCLEX PN Examination. Both of these texts can be ordered from the website – www.nursinged.com. The comments from Nursing Education Consultants' NCLEX Review Course participants, our clinical students, and other nursing faculty have helped to shape the development of these texts.

JoAnn Zerwekh
Jo Carol Claborn

Table of Contents

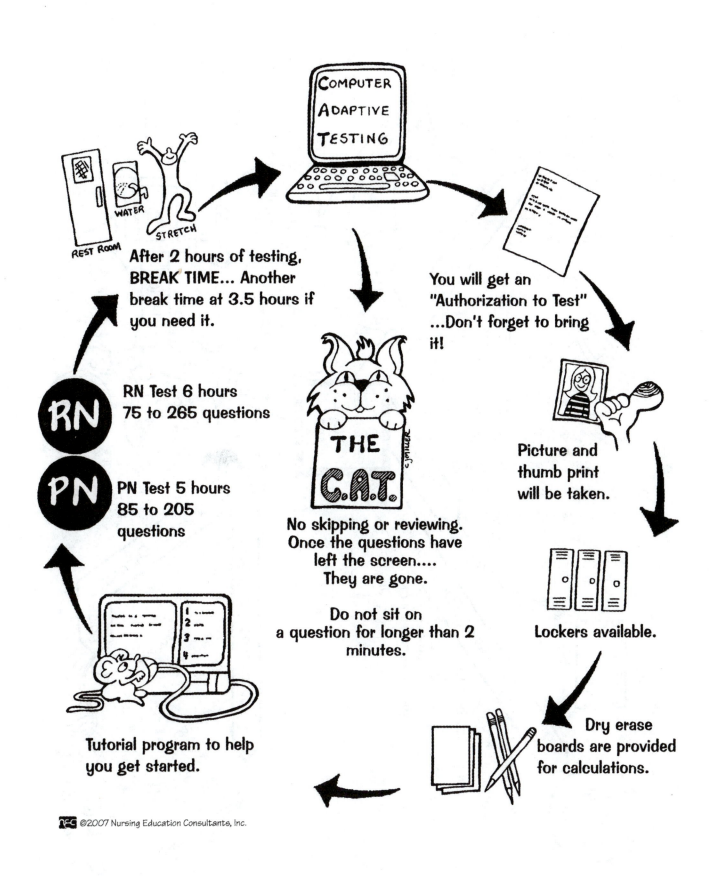

COMPUTER ADAPTIVE TESTING

After 2 hours of testing, **BREAK TIME**... Another break time at 3.5 hours if you need it.

RN Test 6 hours 75 to 265 questions

PN Test 5 hours 85 to 205 questions

THE C.A.T.

No skipping or reviewing. Once the questions have left the screen.... They are gone.

Do not sit on a question for longer than 2 minutes.

You will get an "Authorization to Test" ...Don't forget to bring it!

Picture and thumb print will be taken.

Lockers available.

Dry erase boards are provided for calculations.

Tutorial program to help you get started.

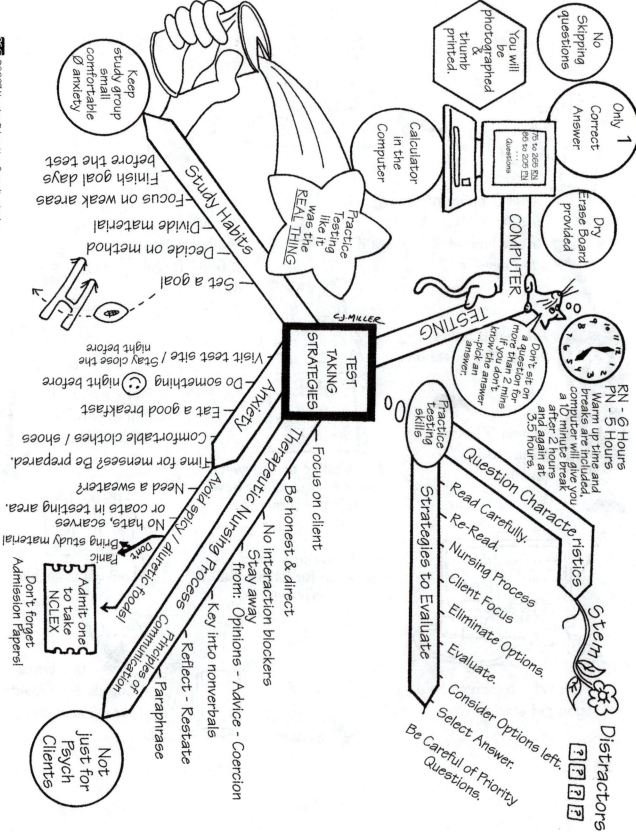

TEST TAKING STRATEGIES

Study Habits
- Keep study group small comfortable Ø anxiety
- Finish goal days before the test
- Focus on weak areas
- Divide material
- Decide on method
- Set a goal
- Practice Testing like it was the REAL THING

Anxiety
- Visit test site / Stay close the night before
- Do something ☺ night before
- Eat a good breakfast
- Comfortable clothes / shoes
- Time for menses? Be prepared.
- Need a sweater?
- No hats, scarves or coats in testing area.
- Bring study material
- Don't Panic
- Admit one to take NCLEX
- Don't forget Admission Papers!
- Avoid spicy / diuretic foods!

Therapeutic Nursing Process
- Focus on client
- Be honest & direct
- No interaction blockers
- Stay away from: Opinions - Advice - Coercion
- Key into nonverbals
- Reflect - Restate
- Paraphrase
- Principles of Communication
- Not just for Psych Clients

COMPUTER
- No Skipping questions
- You will be photographed & thumb printed.
- Only 1 Correct Answer
- Calculator in the Computer
- 75 to 265 RN / 85 to 205 PN Questions
- Dry Erase Board provided

TESTING
- Practice testing skills
- Warm up time and breaks are included, computer will give you a 10 minute break after 2 hours and again at 3.5 hours.
- Don't sit on a question for more than 2 mins — if you don't know the answer...pick an answer.
- RN - 6 Hours
- PN - 5 Hours

Question Characteristics

Strategies to Evaluate
- Read Carefully.
- Re-Read.
- Nursing Process
- Client Focus
- Eliminate Options
- Evaluate.
- Consider Options left.
- Select Answer.
- Be Careful of Priority Questions.

Stem

Distractors
[?] [?] [?]

C.J. MILLER

Maslow's Hiearchy of Basic Human Needs

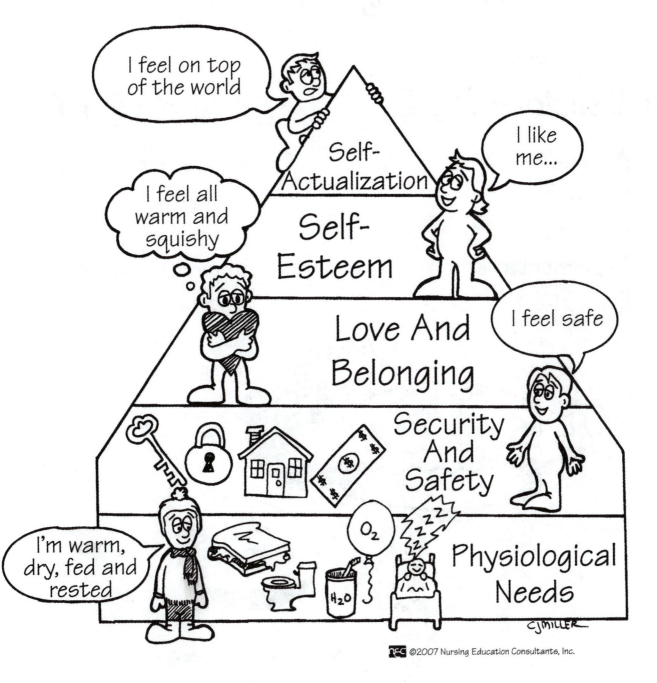

3

Steps in the Nursing Process

A Delicious P I E:

Assessment
Diagnosis
Planning
Implementation
Evaluation

An Apple P I E:

Assessment
Analysis
Planning
Implementation
Evaluation

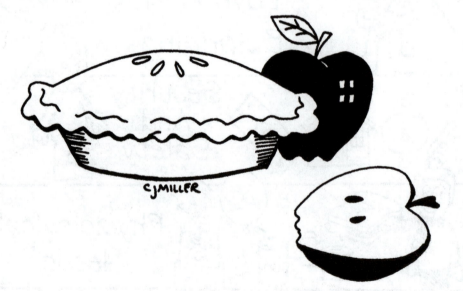

CJMILLER

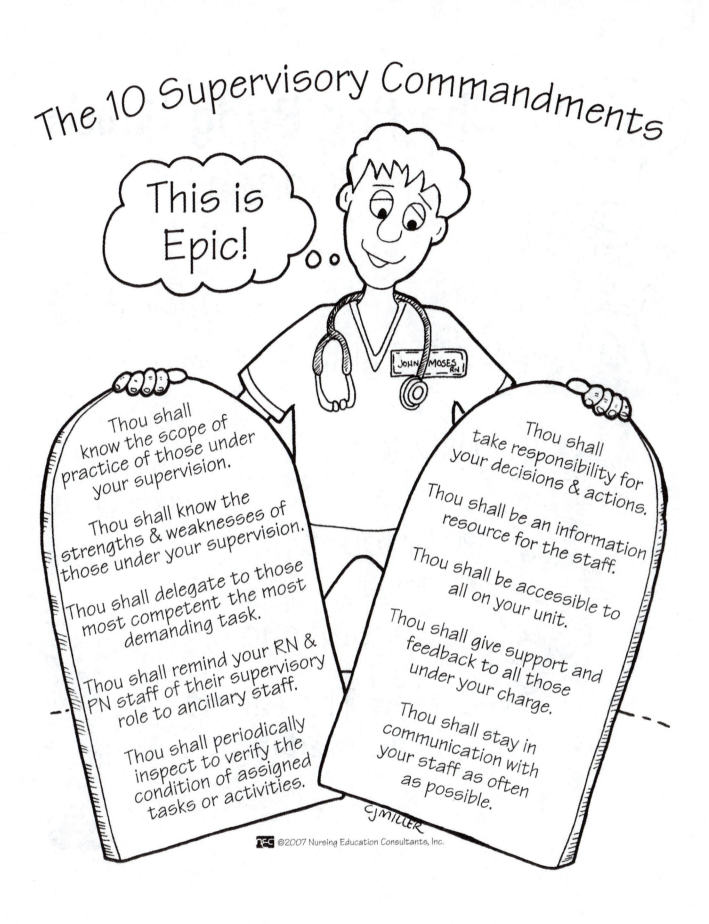

The 10 Supervisory Commandments

This is Epic!

Thou shall know the scope of practice of those under your supervision.

Thou shall know the strengths & weaknesses of those under your supervision.

Thou shall delegate to those most competent the most demanding task.

Thou shall remind your RN & PN staff of their supervisory role to ancillary staff.

Thou shall periodically inspect to verify the condition of assigned tasks or activities.

Thou shall take responsibility for your decisions & actions.

Thou shall be an information resource for the staff.

Thou shall be accessible to all on your unit.

Thou shall give support and feedback to all those under your charge.

Thou shall stay in communication with your staff as often as possible.

©2007 Nursing Education Consultants, Inc.

Charting Body Fluids
"Coach"

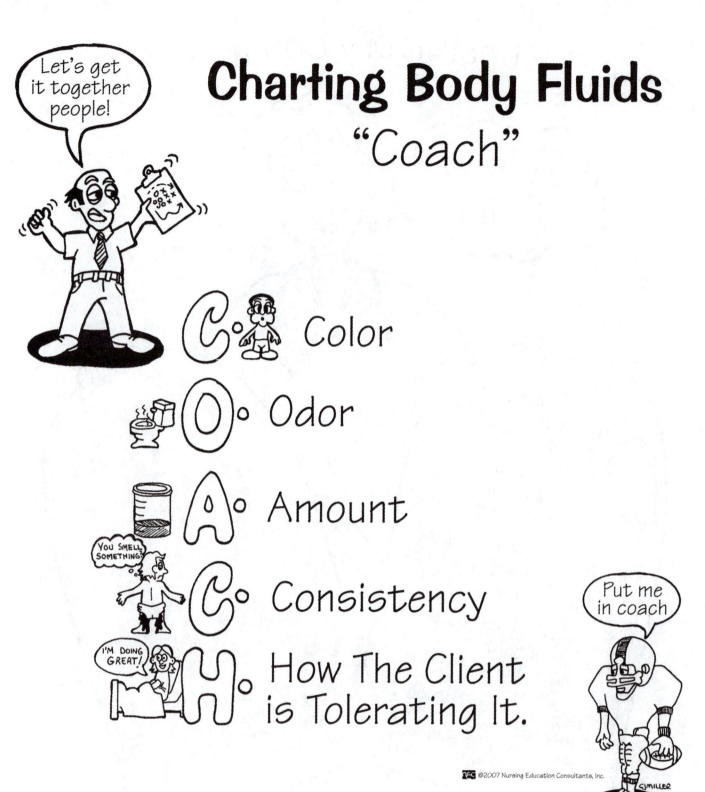

C° Color

O° Odor

A° Amount

C° Consistency

H° How The Client is Tolerating It.

©2007 Nursing Education Consultants, Inc.

CARE OF THE CHRONICALLY ILL CHILD

Focus on child's developmental age vs. chronological age.

Assist child/family to return to normal pattern of living.

Promote child's maximum level of growth and development.

Assess family response to child's illness.

Determine how child is/was cared for at home.

Involve family in care.

Encourage self-care.

Maintain routine if possible.

CJMILLER

Nursing Diagnosis:
- Altered growth and development
- Risk for altered family process
- Anxiety / fear related to test / procedure
- Risk for injury
- Diversional activity deficit
- Impaired social interaction
- Self-care deficit
- Body image disturbance

7

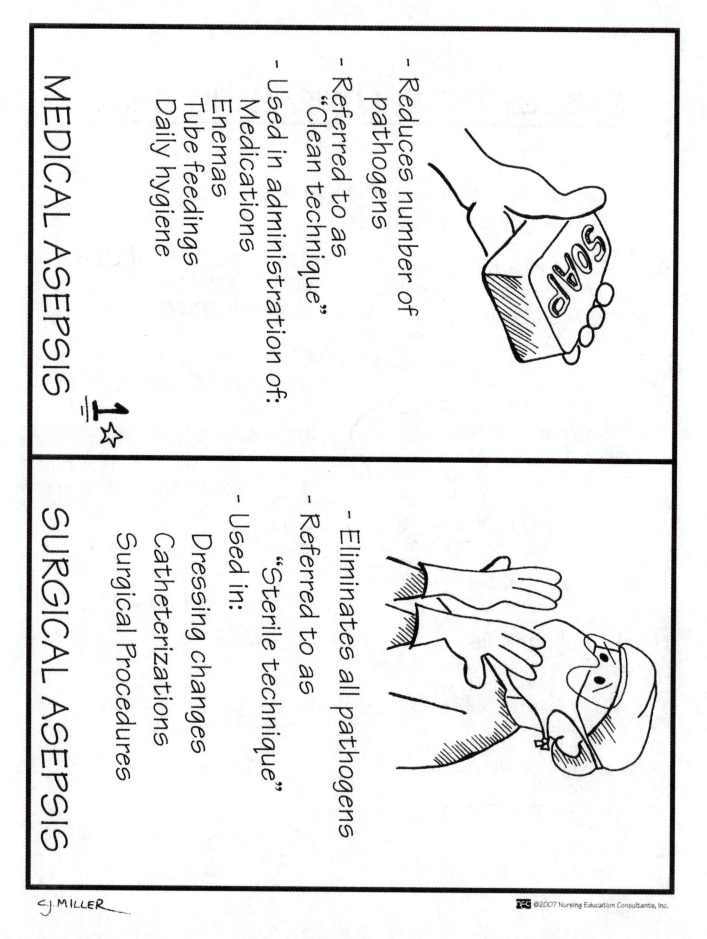

MEDICAL ASEPSIS $\frac{1}{☆}$

- Reduces number of pathogens
- Referred to as "Clean technique"
- Used in administration of:
  Medications
  Enemas
  Tube feedings
  Daily hygiene

SURGICAL ASEPSIS

- Eliminates all pathogens
- Referred to as "Sterile technique"
- Used in:
  Dressing changes
  Catheterizations
  Surgical Procedures

C.J. MILLER

@2007 Nursing Education Consultants, Inc.

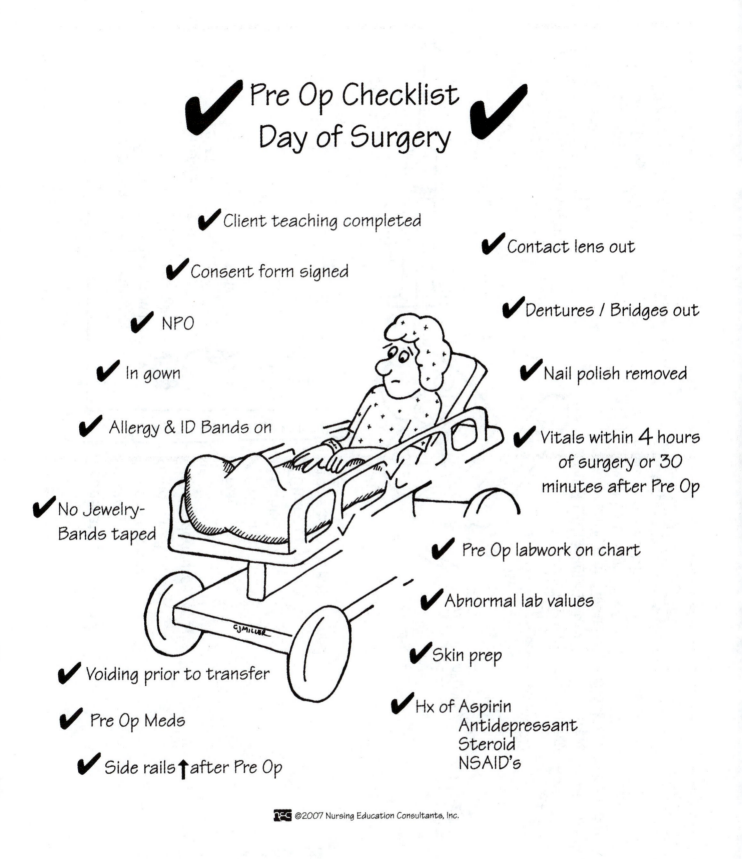

Pre Op Checklist
Day of Surgery

✔ Client teaching completed

✔ Consent form signed

✔ NPO

✔ In gown

✔ Allergy & ID Bands on

✔ No Jewelry-
Bands taped

✔ Voiding prior to transfer

✔ Pre Op Meds

✔ Side rails ↑ after Pre Op

✔ Contact lens out

✔ Dentures / Bridges out

✔ Nail polish removed

✔ Vitals within 4 hours
of surgery or 30
minutes after Pre Op

✔ Pre Op labwork on chart

✔ Abnormal lab values

✔ Skin prep

✔ Hx of Aspirin
Antidepressant
Steroid
NSAID's

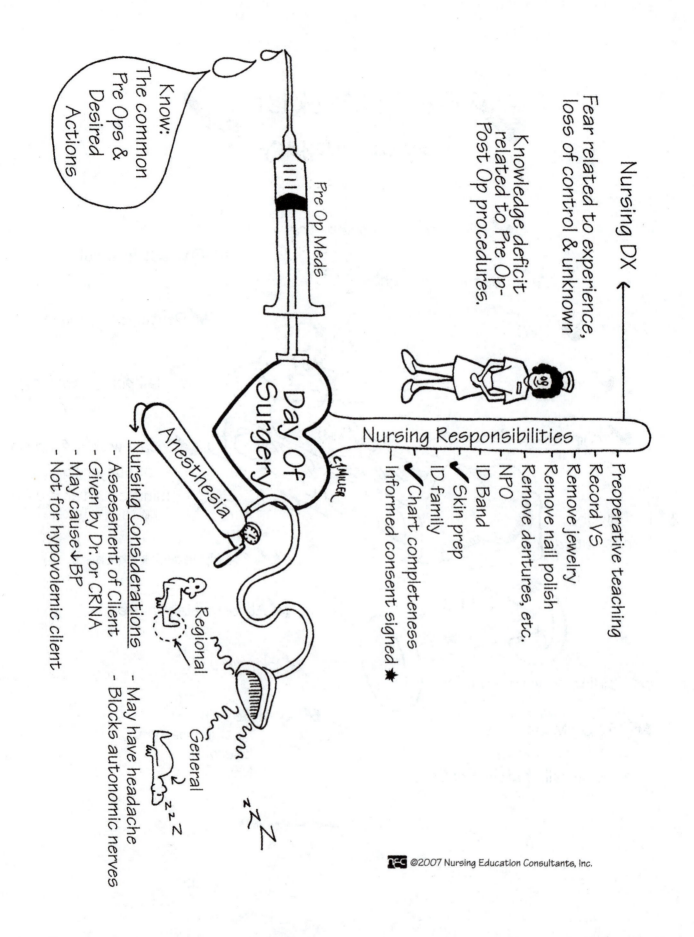

Nursing DX

Fear related to experience,
loss of control & unknown

Knowledge deficit
related to Pre Op-
Post Op procedures.

Know:
The common
Pre Ops &
Desired
Actions

Pre Op Meds

Day Of
Surgery

Nursing Responsibilities

- Preoperative teaching
- Record VS
- Remove jewelry
- Remove nail polish
- Remove dentures, etc.
- NPO
- ID Band
- ID family
- Skin prep
- Chart completeness
- Informed consent signed ✸

Anesthesia

Nursing Considerations

- Assessment of Client
- Given by Dr. or CRNA
- May cause ↓BP
- Not for hypovolemic client

Regional
- May have headache
- Blocks autonomic nerves

General

C.J. MILLER

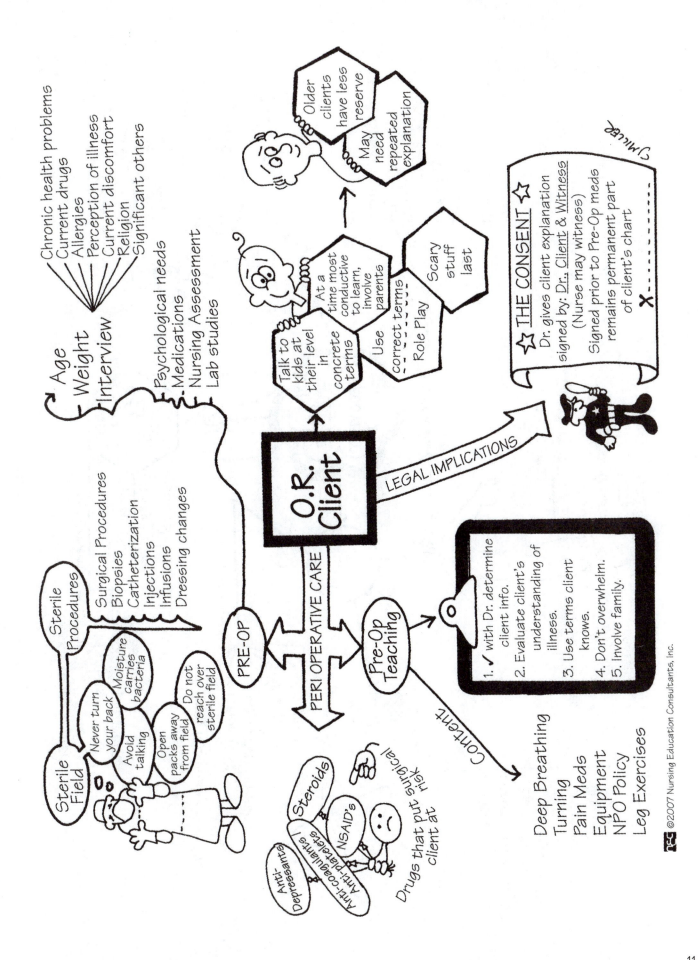

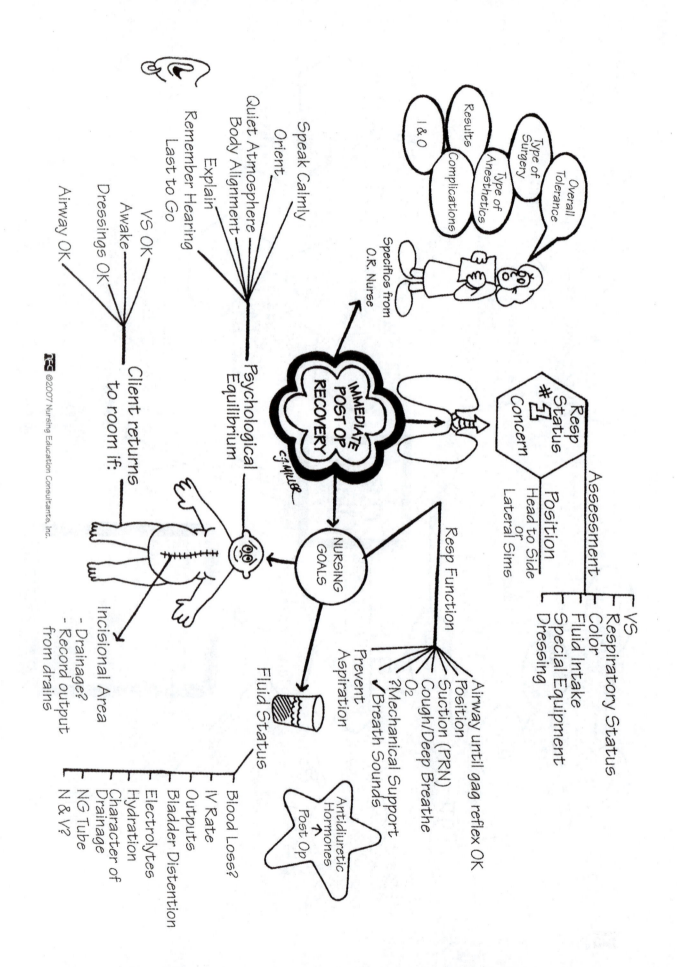

IMMEDIATE POST OP RECOVERY

Specifics from O.R. Nurse
- Type of Surgery
- Type of Anesthetics
- Results
- Complications
- I & O
- Overall Tolerance

Assessment
- VS
- Respiratory Status
- Color
- Fluid Intake
- Special Equipment
- Dressing

Resp Status #1 Concern

Position
- Head to Side or Lateral Sims

Resp Function
- Airway until gag reflex OK
- Position
- Suction (PRN)
- Cough/Deep Breathe
- O_2
- ?Mechanical Support
- ✓Breath Sounds

Prevent Aspiration

Antidiuretic Hormones → Post Op

NURSING GOALS

Fluid Status
- Blood Loss?
- IV Rate
- Outputs
- Bladder Distention
- Electrolytes
- Hydration
- Character of Drainage
- NG Tube
- N & V?

Incisional Area
- Drainage?
- Record output from drains

Psychological Equilibrium
- Speak Calmly
- Orient
- Quiet Atmosphere
- Body Alignment
- Explain
- Remember Hearing
- Last to Go

Client returns to room if:
- VS OK
- Awake
- Dressings OK
- Airway OK

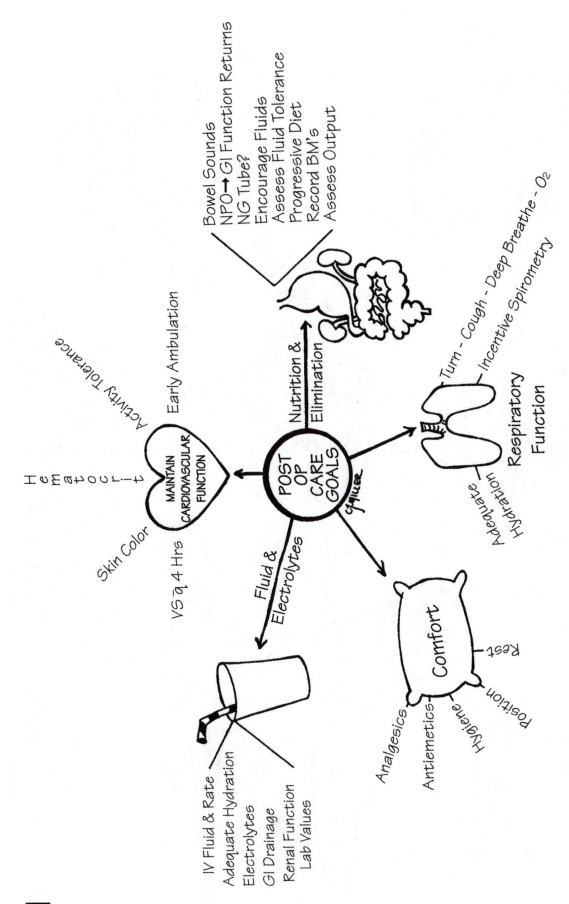

Bowel Sounds
NPO → GI Function Returns
NG Tube?
Encourage Fluids
Assess Fluid Tolerance
Progressive Diet
Record BM's
Assess Output

Nutrition &
Elimination

Early Ambulation

Activity Tolerance

MAINTAIN
CARDIOVASCULAR
FUNCTION

Hematocrit

Skin Color

VS q̄ 4 Hrs

POST
OP
CARE
GOALS

Turn - Cough - Deep Breathe - O₂

Incentive Spirometry

Respiratory
Function

Adequate Hydration

Fluid &
Electrolytes

IV Fluid & Rate
Adequate Hydration
Electrolytes
GI Drainage
Renal Function
Lab Values

Comfort

Rest

Position

Hygiene

Antiemetics

Analgesics

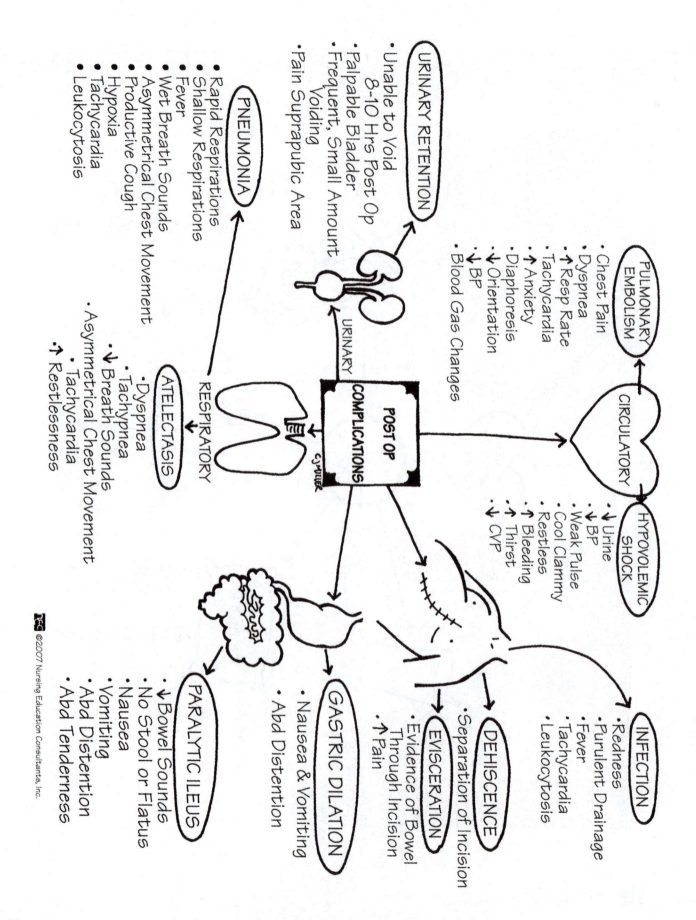

POST OP COMPLICATIONS

URINARY

URINARY RETENTION
- Unable to Void
- 8-10 Hrs Post Op
- Palpable Bladder
- Frequent, Small Amount Voiding
- Pain Suprapubic Area

RESPIRATORY

PNEUMONIA
- Rapid Respirations
- Shallow Respirations
- Fever
- Wet Breath Sounds
- Asymmetrical Chest Movement
- Productive Cough
- Hypoxia
- Tachycardia
- Leukocytosis

ATELECTASIS
- Dyspnea
- ↑ Tachypnea
- ↓ Breath Sounds
- Asymmetrical Chest Movement
- ↑ Tachycardia
- ↑ Restlessness

CIRCULATORY

PULMONARY EMBOLISM
- Chest Pain
- Dyspnea
- ↑ Resp Rate
- Tachycardia
- Anxiety
- Diaphoresis
- ↓ Orientation
- ↓ BP
- Blood Gas Changes

HYPOVOLEMIC SHOCK
- ↓ Urine
- ↓ BP
- ↑ Weak Pulse
- Restless
- Cool Clammy
- ↑ Bleeding
- ↑ Thirst
- ↓ CVP

PARALYTIC ILEUS
- ↓ Bowel Sounds
- No Stool or Flatus
- Nausea
- Vomiting
- Abd Distention
- Abd Tenderness

GASTRIC DILATION
- Nausea & Vomiting
- Abd Distention

EVISCERATION
- Evidence of Bowel Through Incision
- ↑ Pain

DEHISCENCE
- Separation of Incision

INFECTION
- Redness
- Purulent Drainage
- Fever
- Tachycardia
- Leukocytosis

DEHISCENCE / EVISCERATION

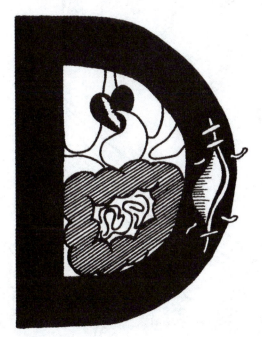

Dehiscence

Separation or splitting open of layers of a surgical wound

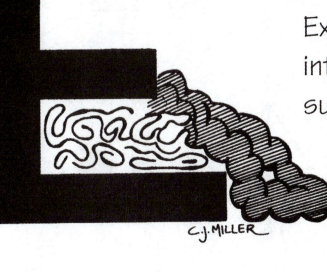

C.J. MILLER

Evisceration

Extrusion of viscera or intestine through a surgical wound

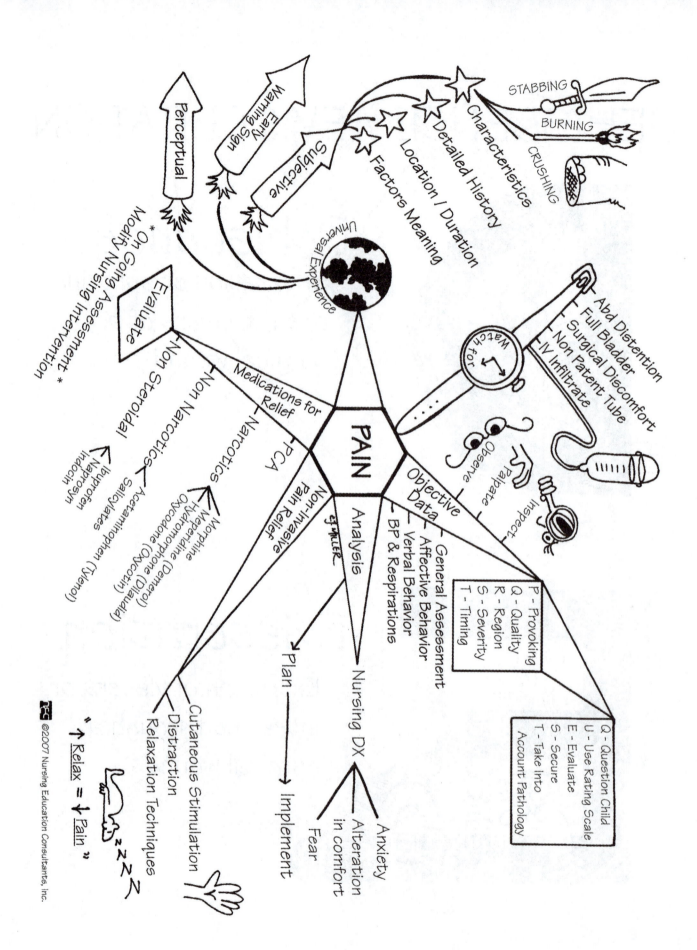

PAIN

Characteristics
STABBING
BURNING
CRUSHING

Subjective
Early Warning Sign
Perceptual

On Going Nursing Assessment *
Modify Nursing Intervention *

Evaluate

Detailed History
Location / Duration
Factors Meaning

Universal Experience

Medications for Relief

Non Steroidal
Ibuprofen (Motrin)
Naprosyn
Salicylates
Acetaminophen (Tylenol)

Non Narcotics

Narcotics
Morphine
Meperidine (Demerol)
Hydromorphone (Dilaudid)
Oxycodone (Oxycontin)

PCA

Non-Invasive Pain Relief

Analysis
by MILLER

Cutaneous Stimulation
Distraction
Relaxation Techniques

Plan

Implement

Nursing DX
Anxiety
Alteration in comfort
Fear

BP & Respirations
Verbal Behavior
Affective Behavior
General Assessment

Objective Data

Watch for

Abd Distention
Full Bladder
Surgical Discomfort
Non Patent Tube
IV Infiltrate

Observe
Palpate
Inspect

P - Provoking
Q - Quality
R - Region
S - Severity
T - Timing

Q - Question Child
U - Use Rating Scale
E - Evaluate
S - Secure
T - Take Into Account Pathology

"↑ Relax = ↓ Pain"
zzz

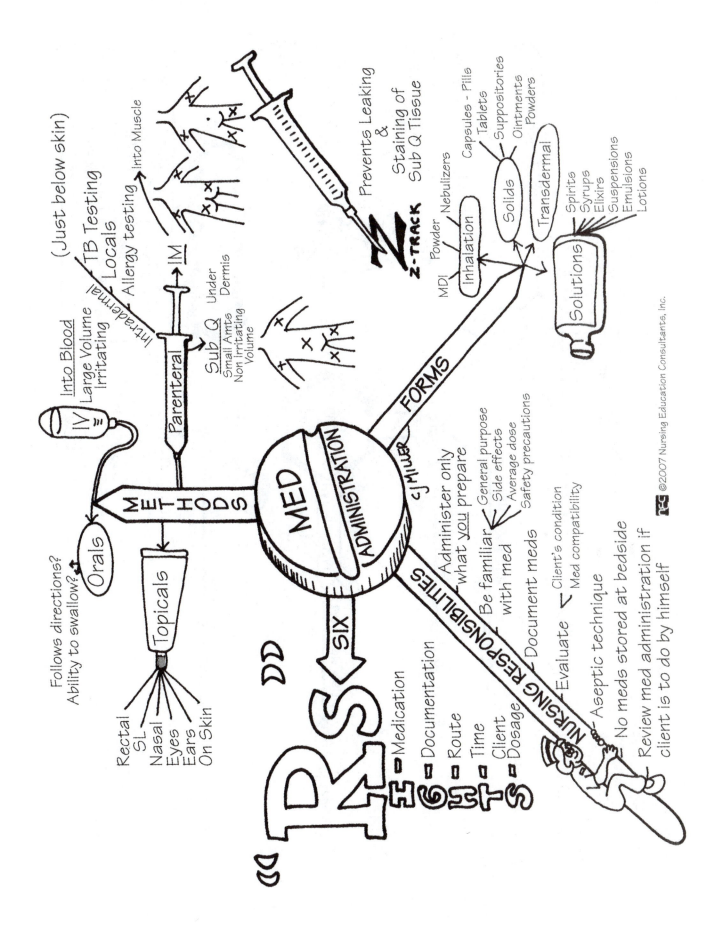

MED ADMINISTRATION

© J. Miller

METHODS

Orals
- Follows directions?
- Ability to swallow?

Topicals
- Rectal
- SL
- Nasal
- Eyes
- Ears
- On Skin

IV — Into Blood
- Large Volume
- Irritating

Parenteral

Intradermal (Just below skin)
- TB Testing
- Locals
- Allergy testing

IM — Into Muscle

Sub Q — Under Dermis
- Small Amts
- Non Irritating Volume

Z-TRACK
Prevents Leaking & Staining of Sub Q Tissue

FORMS

Inhalation
- MDI
- Powder
- Nebulizers

Solids
- Capsules – Pills
- Tablets
- Suppositories
- Ointments
- Powders

Transdermal

Solutions
- Spirits
- Syrups
- Elixirs
- Suspensions
- Emulsions
- Lotions

SIX RRS
- R = Medication
- R = Documentation
- R = Route
- R = Time
- R = Client
- R = Dosage

NURSING RESPONSIBILITIES
- Administer only what you prepare
- Be familiar with med
  - General purpose
  - Side effects
  - Average dose
  - Safety precautions
- Document meds
- Evaluate
  - Client's condition
  - Med compatibility
- Aseptic technique
- No meds stored at bedside
- Review med administration if client is to do by himself

© 2007 Nursing Education Consultants, Inc.

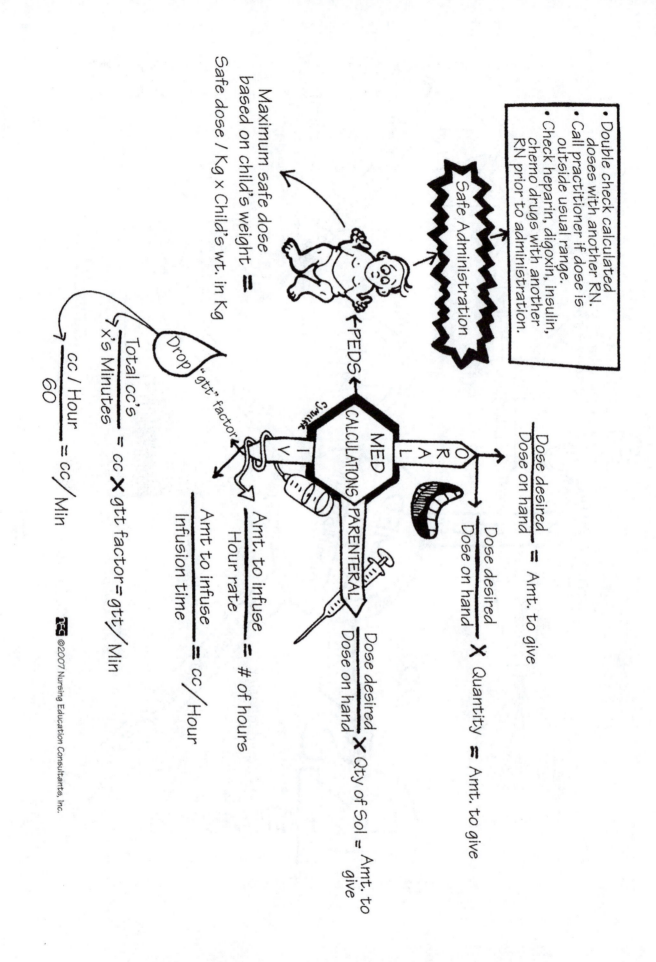

Safe Administration

- Double check calculated doses with another RN.
- Call practitioner if dose is outside usual range.
- Check heparin, digoxin, insulin, chemo drugs with another RN prior to administration.

PEDS

Maximum safe dose based on child's weight =
Safe dose / Kg x Child's wt. in Kg

MED CALCULATIONS

ORAL

$$\frac{\text{Dose desired}}{\text{Dose on hand}} = \text{Amt. to give}$$

$$\frac{\text{Dose desired}}{\text{Dose on hand}} \times \text{Quantity} = \text{Amt. to give}$$

PARENTERAL

$$\frac{\text{Dose desired}}{\text{Dose on hand}} \times \text{Qty of Sol} = \text{Amt. to give}$$

IV

Drop "gtt" factor

$$\frac{\text{Total cc's}}{\text{x's Minutes}} = \text{cc} \times \text{gtt factor} = \text{gtt/Min}$$

$$\frac{\text{cc / Hour}}{60} = \text{cc/Min}$$

$$\frac{\text{Amt. to infuse}}{\text{Hour rate}} = \text{# of hours}$$

$$\frac{\text{Amt. to infuse}}{\text{Infusion time}} = \text{cc/Hour}$$

ATROPINE OVERDOSE

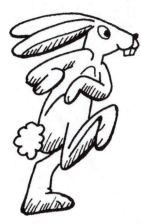

Hot as a Hare
($\uparrow$ temperature)

Mad as a Hatter
(confusion, delirium)

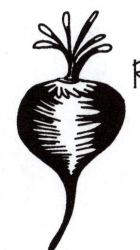

Red as a Beet
(flushed face)

Dry as a Bone
(decreased secretions, thirsty)

From: Robert W. Malone, RN

EAR DROPS ADMINISTRATION

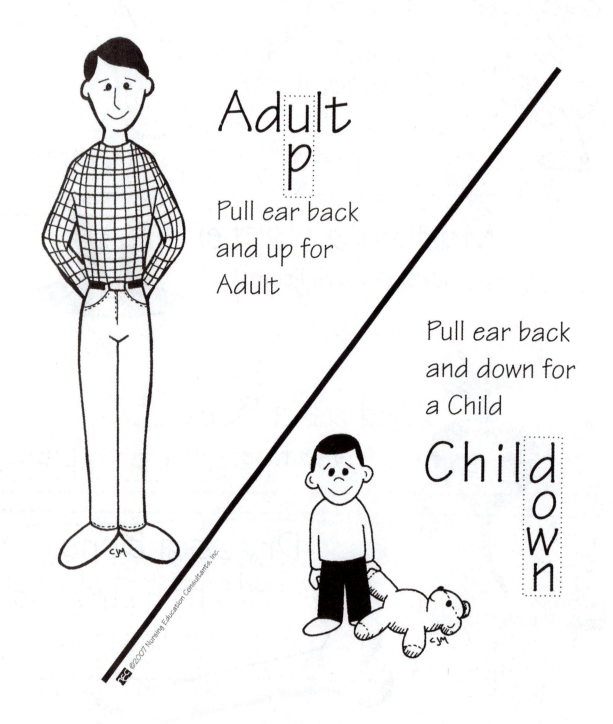

Adult
p
Pull ear back
and up for
Adult

Pull ear back
and down for
a Child

Child
down

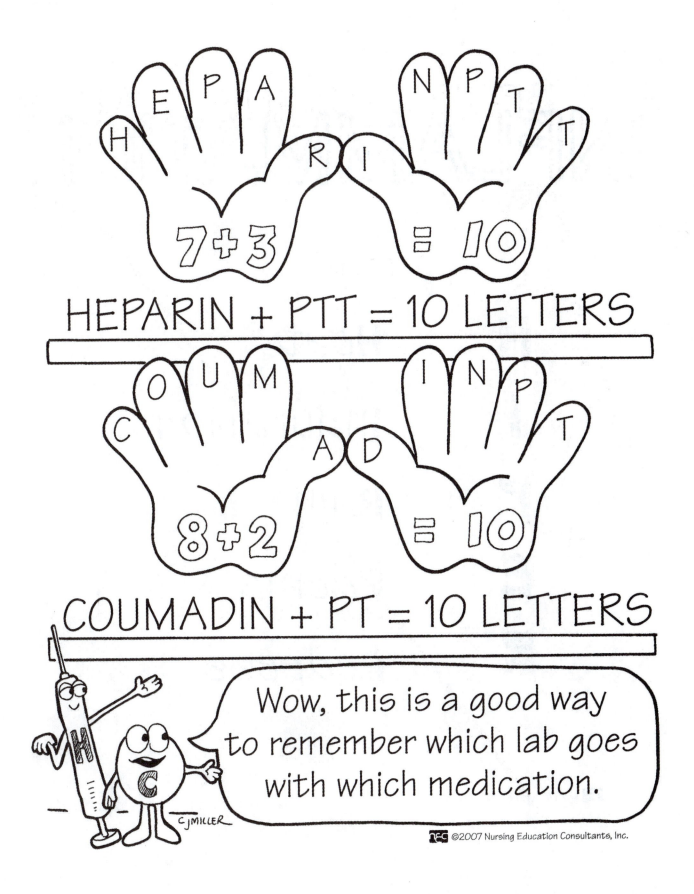

HEPARIN + PTT = 10 LETTERS

COUMADIN + PT = 10 LETTERS

Wow, this is a good way to remember which lab goes with which medication.

INFLAMMATION

H **H**eat

I **I**nduration

P **P**ain

E **E**dema

R **R**edness

Adapted from Dolores Graceffa, RN, MS

RESPIRATORY ACIDOSIS

- Hypoventilation → Hypoxia

- Rapid, Shallow Respirations

- ↓ BP with Vasodilation

- Dyspnea

- Headache

- Hyperkalemia

- Dysrhythmias (↑K)

- Drowsiness, Dizziness, Disorientation

- Muscle Weakness, Hyperreflexia

- Causes: ↓Respiratory Stimuli (Anesthesia, Drug Overdose) COPD Pneumonia Atelectasis

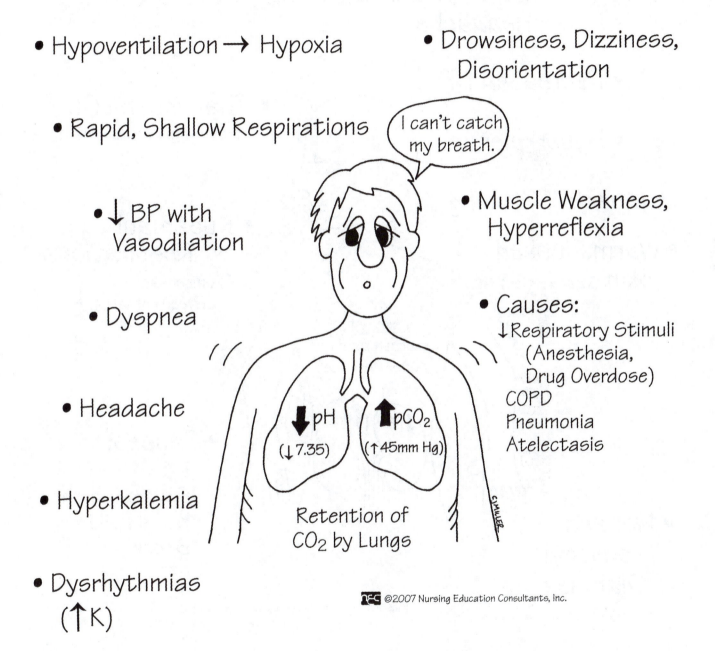

I can't catch my breath.

↓pH (↓7.35)   ↑pCO$_2$ (↑45mm Hg)

Retention of CO$_2$ by Lungs

METABOLIC ACIDOSIS

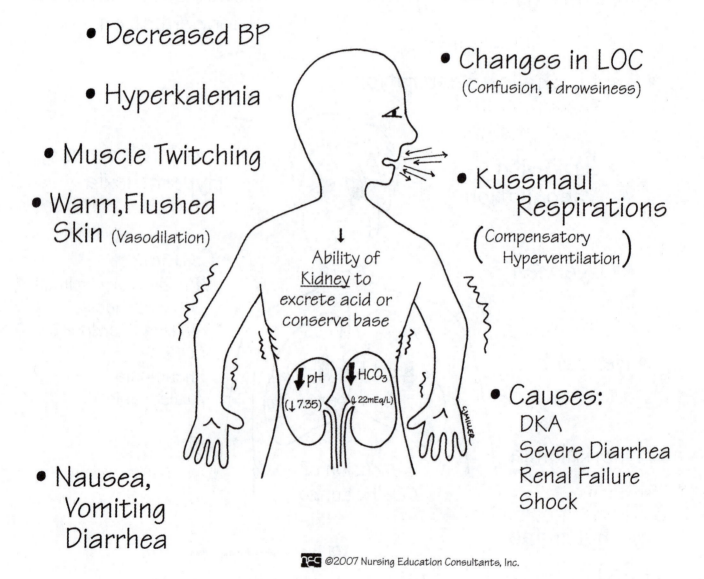

- Headache
- Decreased BP
- Hyperkalemia
- Muscle Twitching
- Warm, Flushed Skin (Vasodilation)
- Nausea, Vomiting Diarrhea

- Changes in LOC (Confusion, ↑drowsiness)
- Kussmaul Respirations (Compensatory Hyperventilation)
- Causes:
  DKA
  Severe Diarrhea
  Renal Failure
  Shock

↓
Ability of Kidney to excrete acid or conserve base

↓pH (↓7.35)   ↓HCO₃ (↓22mEq/L)

RESPIRATORY ALKALOSIS

- Seizures

- Deep, Rapid Breathing

- Hyperventilation

- Tachycardia

- ↓ or Normal BP

- Hypokalemia

- Numbness & Tingling of Extremities

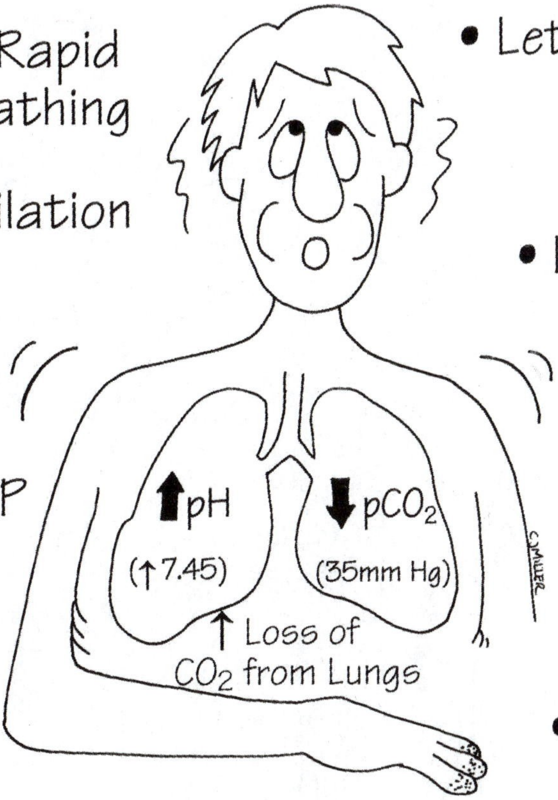

- Lethargy & Confusion

- Light Headedness

- Nausea, Vomiting

- Causes:
  Hyperventilation
  (Anxiety, PE, Fear)
  Mechanical Ventilation

↑pH
(↑7.45)

↓pCO$_2$
(35mm Hg)

↑ Loss of CO$_2$ from Lungs

METABOLIC ALKALOSIS

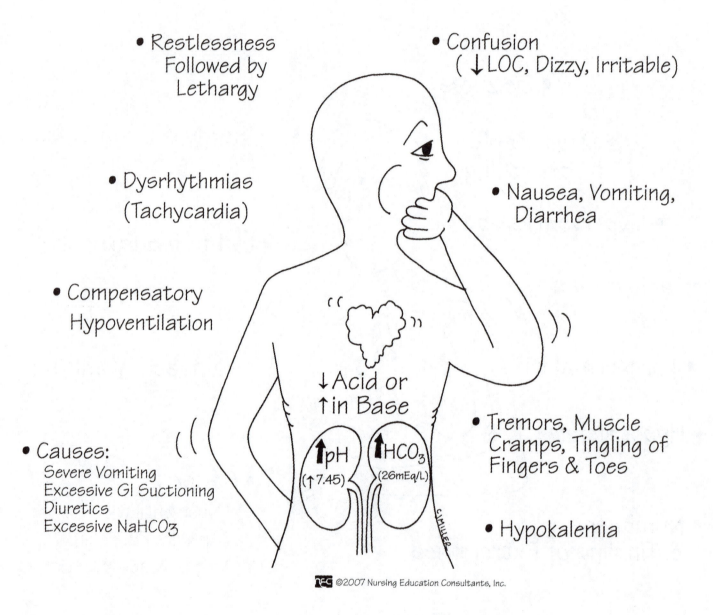

- Restlessness Followed by Lethargy

- Confusion (↓LOC, Dizzy, Irritable)

- Dysrhythmias (Tachycardia)

- Nausea, Vomiting, Diarrhea

- Compensatory Hypoventilation

↓Acid or ↑in Base

↑pH (↑7.45) ↑HCO₃ (26mEq/L)

- Tremors, Muscle Cramps, Tingling of Fingers & Toes

- Causes:
  Severe Vomiting
  Excessive GI Suctioning
  Diuretics
  Excessive NaHCO₃

- Hypokalemia

C.MILLER

©2007 Nursing Education Consultants, Inc.

ACID BASE MNEMONIC
(ROME)

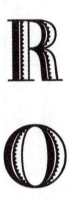

Respiratory

Opposite

pH ↑ PCO_2 ↓   Alkalosis

pH ↓ PCO_2 ↑   Acidosis

Metabolic

Equal

pH ↑ HCO_3 ↑   Alkalosis

pH ↓ HCO_3 ↓   Acidosis

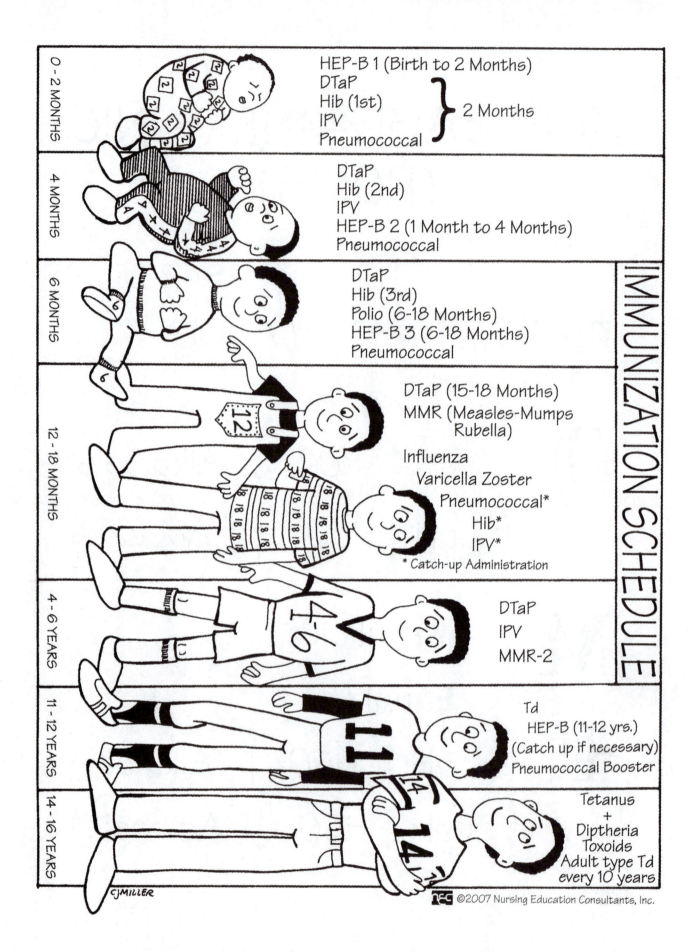

IMMUNIZATION SCHEDULE

0 - 2 MONTHS
HEP-B 1 (Birth to 2 Months)
DTaP
Hib (1st)
IPV
Pneumococcal
} 2 Months

4 MONTHS
DTaP
Hib (2nd)
IPV
HEP-B 2 (1 Month to 4 Months)
Pneumococcal

6 MONTHS
DTaP
Hib (3rd)
Polio (6-18 Months)
HEP-B 3 (6-18 Months)
Pneumococcal

12 - 18 MONTHS
DTaP (15-18 Months)
MMR (Measles-Mumps Rubella)
Influenza
Varicella Zoster
Pneumococcal*
Hib*
IPV*
* Catch-up Administration

4 - 6 YEARS
DTaP
IPV
MMR-2

11 - 12 YEARS
Td
HEP-B (11-12 yrs.)
(Catch up if necessary)
Pneumococcal Booster

14 - 16 YEARS
Tetanus
+
Diptheria
Toxoids
Adult type Td
every 10 years

CJMILLER ©2007 Nursing Education Consultants, Inc.

CLINICAL MANIFESTATION OF AIDS

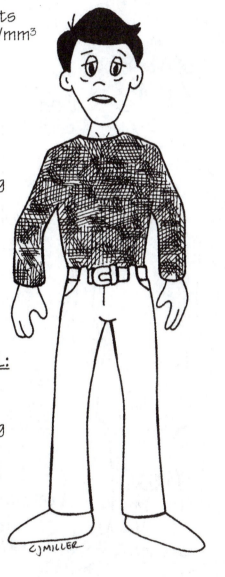

IMMUNOLOGIC:
- Low white cell counts
  CDT_4 count < 200/mm³
- Opportunistic
  Infections
- Lymphadenopathy
- Fatigue

INTEGUMENTARY:
- Poor Wound Healing
- Skin Lesions
- Night Sweats

RESPIRATORY:
- Cough
- SOB

GASTROINTESTINAL:
- Diarrhea
- Weight Loss
- Nausea/Vomiting

CENTRAL NERVOUS SYSTEM:
- Confusion
- Dementia
- Headache
- Visual Changes
- Personality Changes
- Pain
- Seizures

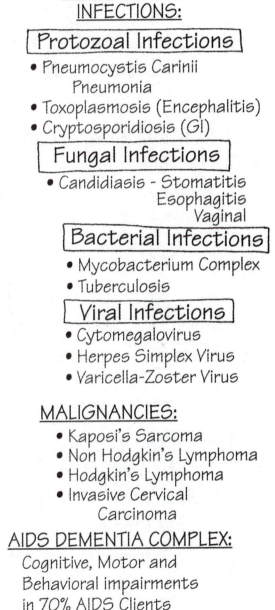

OPPORTUNISTIC INFECTIONS:

Protozoal Infections
- Pneumocystis Carinii
  Pneumonia
- Toxoplasmosis (Encephalitis)
- Cryptosporidiosis (GI)

Fungal Infections
- Candidiasis - Stomatitis
  Esophagitis
  Vaginal

Bacterial Infections
- Mycobacterium Complex
- Tuberculosis

Viral Infections
- Cytomegalovirus
- Herpes Simplex Virus
- Varicella-Zoster Virus

MALIGNANCIES:
- Kaposi's Sarcoma
- Non Hodgkin's Lymphoma
- Hodgkin's Lymphoma
- Invasive Cervical
  Carcinoma

AIDS DEMENTIA COMPLEX:
Cognitive, Motor and
Behavioral impairments
in 70% AIDS Clients

CJMILLER

nec ©2007 Nursing Education Consultants, Inc.

AIDS: PREVENTION OF TRANSMISSION IN THE HEALTH CARE SETTING

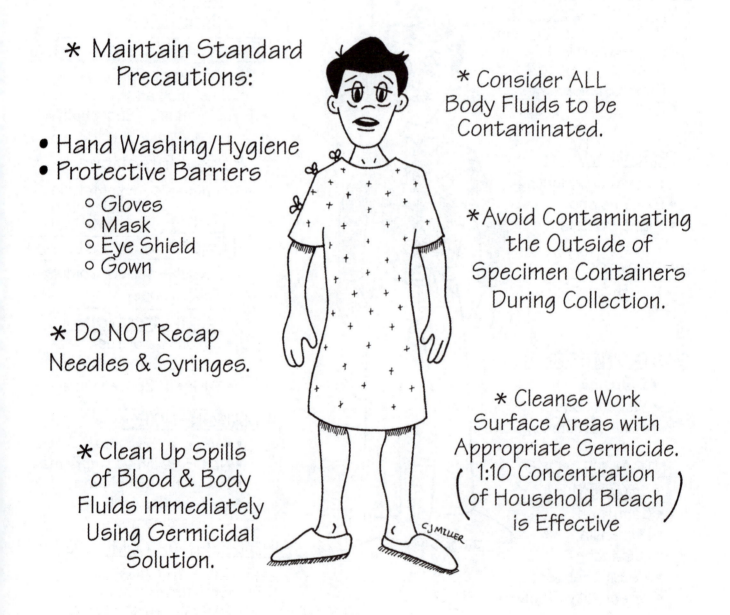

* Maintain Standard Precautions:

- Hand Washing/Hygiene
- Protective Barriers
  - Gloves
  - Mask
  - Eye Shield
  - Gown

* Do NOT Recap Needles & Syringes.

* Clean Up Spills of Blood & Body Fluids Immediately Using Germicidal Solution.

* Consider ALL Body Fluids to be Contaminated.

* Avoid Contaminating the Outside of Specimen Containers During Collection.

* Cleanse Work Surface Areas with Appropriate Germicide. (1:10 Concentration of Household Bleach) is Effective

Infectious Mononucleosis
"Mono"

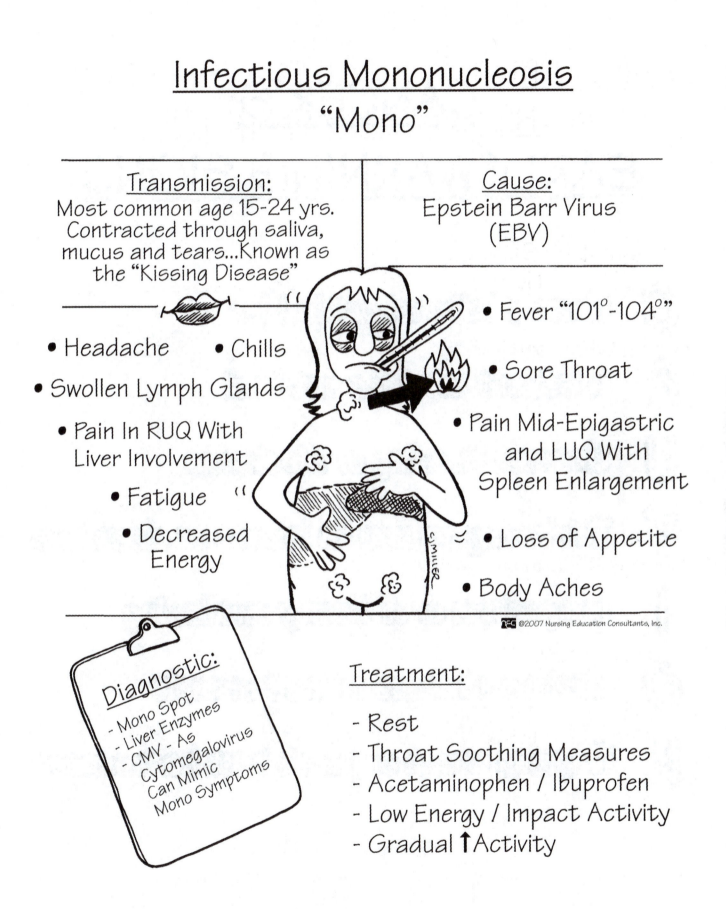

Transmission:
Most common age 15-24 yrs. Contracted through saliva, mucus and tears...Known as the "Kissing Disease"

Cause:
Epstein Barr Virus (EBV)

- Headache
- Chills
- Swollen Lymph Glands
- Pain In RUQ With Liver Involvement
- Fatigue
- Decreased Energy

- Fever "101°-104°"
- Sore Throat
- Pain Mid-Epigastric and LUQ With Spleen Enlargement
- Loss of Appetite
- Body Aches

@2007 Nursing Education Consultants, Inc.

Diagnostic:
- Mono Spot
- Liver Enzymes
- CMV - As Cytomegalovirus Can Mimic Mono Symptoms

Treatment:
- Rest
- Throat Soothing Measures
- Acetaminophen / Ibuprofen
- Low Energy / Impact Activity
- Gradual ↑Activity

31

CANCER'S
EARLY WARNING SIGNS

C Change in bowel or bladder

A A lesion that does not heal

U Unusual bleeding or discharge

T Thickening or lump in breast or elsewhere

I Indigestion or difficulty swallowing

O Obvious changes in wart or mole

N Nagging cough or persistent hoarseness

Reprinted with permission by American Cancer Society, Cancer Facts and Figures, 1992   NEC ©2007 Nursing Education Consultants, Inc.

CANCER

C	**C**omfort
A	**A**ltered Body Image
N	**N**utrition
C	**C**hemotherapy
E	**E**valuate Response to Meds
R	**R**espite for Caretakers

ALTERATIONS OF BODY IMAGE:
FOUR PHASES

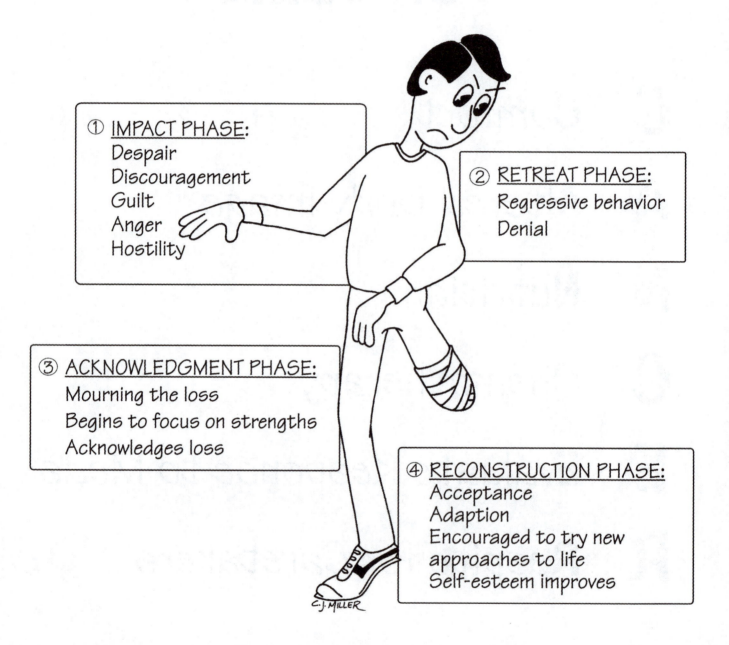

① IMPACT PHASE:
Despair
Discouragement
Guilt
Anger
Hostility

② RETREAT PHASE:
Regressive behavior
Denial

③ ACKNOWLEDGMENT PHASE:
Mourning the loss
Begins to focus on strengths
Acknowledges loss

④ RECONSTRUCTION PHASE:
Acceptance
Adaption
Encouraged to try new
approaches to life
Self-esteem improves

C.J. MILLER

BASIC COMPONENTS
OF A PSYCH ASSESSMENT

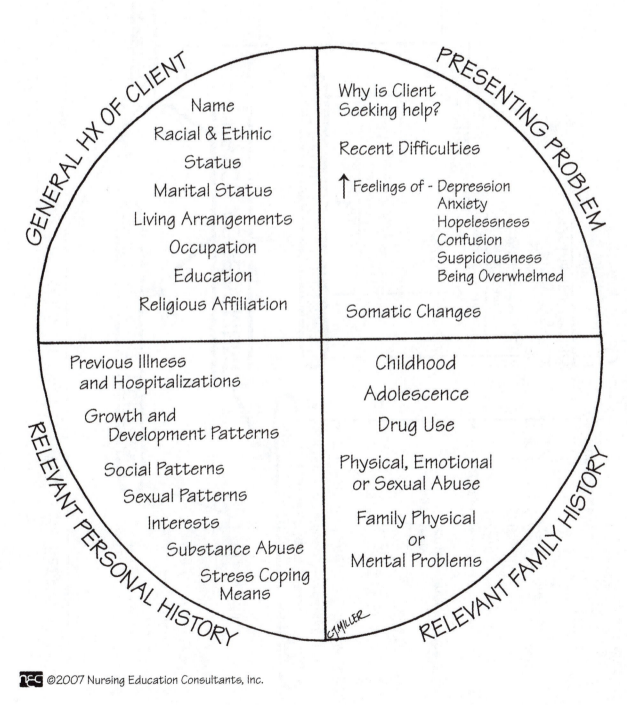

GENERAL HX OF CLIENT

Name
Racial & Ethnic
Status
Marital Status
Living Arrangements
Occupation
Education
Religious Affiliation

PRESENTING PROBLEM

Why is Client
Seeking help?

Recent Difficulties

↑ Feelings of - Depression
Anxiety
Hopelessness
Confusion
Suspiciousness
Being Overwhelmed

Somatic Changes

RELEVANT PERSONAL HISTORY

Previous Illness
and Hospitalizations

Growth and
Development Patterns

Social Patterns
Sexual Patterns
Interests
Substance Abuse
Stress Coping
Means

RELEVANT FAMILY HISTORY

Childhood

Adolescence

Drug Use

Physical, Emotional
or Sexual Abuse

Family Physical
or
Mental Problems

CJMILLER

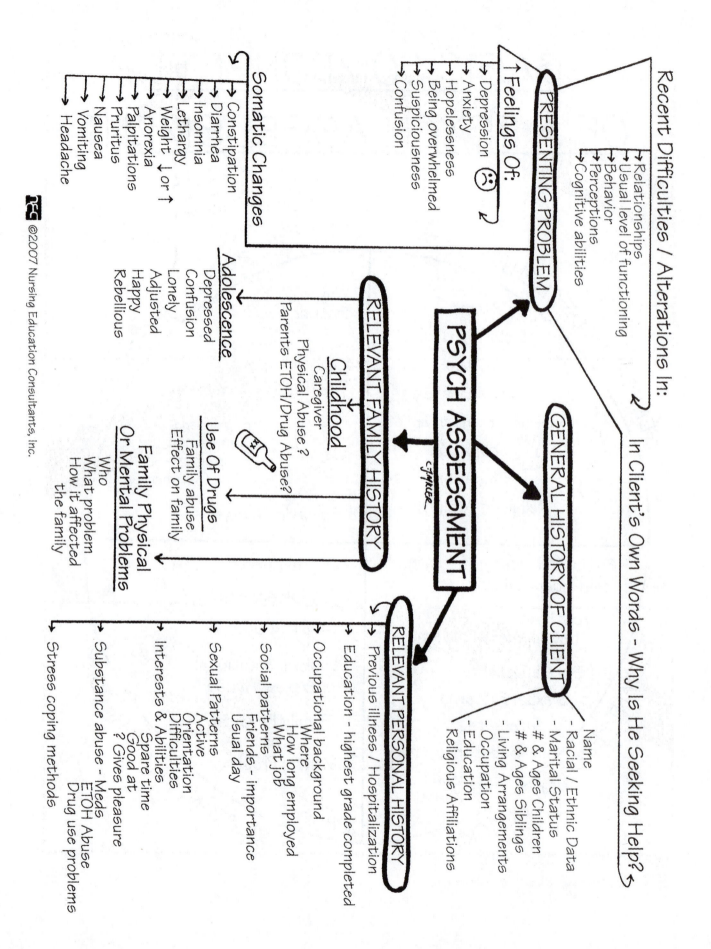

Recent Difficulties / Alterations In:
→ Relationships
→ Usual level of functioning
→ Behavior
→ Perceptions
→ Cognitive abilities

→ Feelings Of:
→ Depression 😞
→ Anxiety
→ Hopelessness
→ Being overwhelmed
→ Suspiciousness
→ Confusion

PRESENTING PROBLEM

Somatic Changes
→ Constipation
→ Diarrhea
→ Insomnia
→ Lethargy
→ Weight ↓ or ↑
→ Anorexia
→ Palpitations
→ Pruritus
→ Nausea
→ Vomiting
→ Headache

RELEVANT FAMILY HISTORY

Adolescence
Depressed
Confusion
Lonely
Adjusted
Happy
Rebellious

Childhood
Caregiver
Physical Abuse ?
Parents ETOH/Drug Abuse?

Use Of Drugs
Family abuse
Effect on family

Family Physical
Or Mental Problems
Who
What problem
How it affected
the family

PSYCH ASSESSMENT
C. Miller

GENERAL HISTORY OF CLIENT
- Name
- Racial / Ethnic Data
- Marital Status
- # & Ages Children
- # & Ages Siblings
- Living Arrangements
- Occupation
- Education
- Religious Affiliations

In Client's Own Words - Why Is He Seeking Help?

RELEVANT PERSONAL HISTORY
Previous illness / Hospitalization
Education - highest grade completed
Occupational background
   Where
   How long employed
   What job
   Usual day
Social patterns
   Friends - importance
Sexual Patterns
   Active
   Orientation
   Difficulties
Interests & Abilities
   Spare time
   Good at
   ? Gives pleasure
Substance abuse - Meds
   ETOH Abuse
   Drug use problems
Stress coping methods

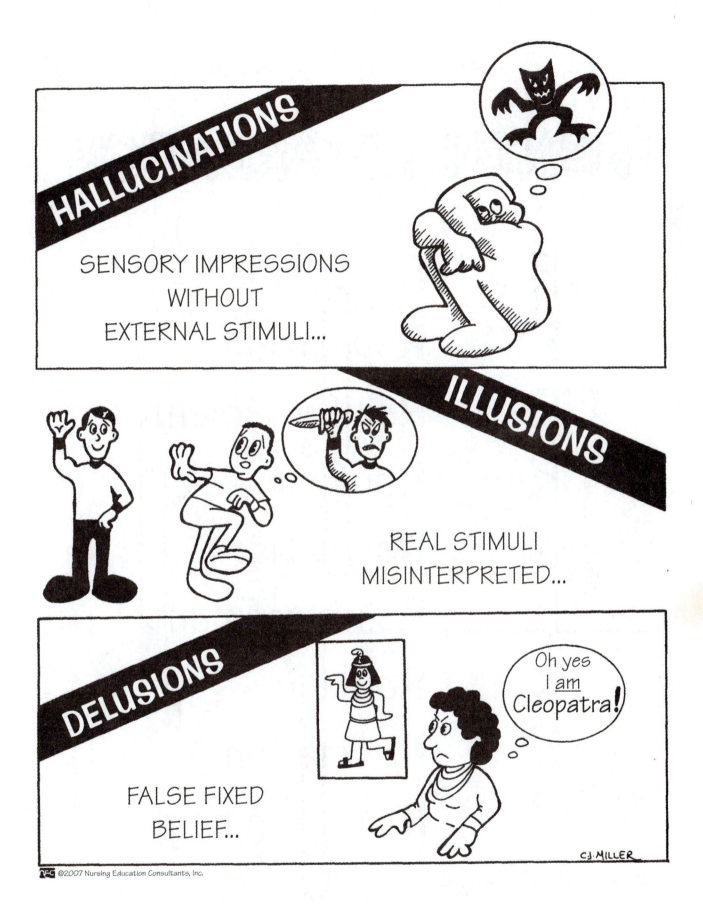

MENTAL RETARDATION

R **R**outine

R **R**epetition

R **R**einforcement

R **R**outine

R **R**epetition

R **R**einforcement

R **R**outine

R **R**epetition

R **R**einforcement

DOWN'S SYNDROME

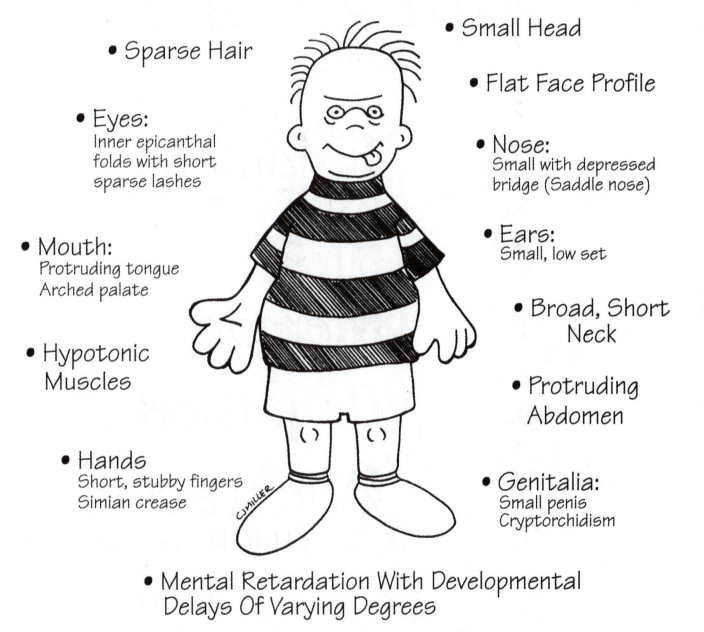

- Sparse Hair

- Eyes:
Inner epicanthal
folds with short
sparse lashes

- Mouth:
Protruding tongue
Arched palate

- Hypotonic
Muscles

- Hands
Short, stubby fingers
Simian crease

- Small Head

- Flat Face Profile

- Nose:
Small with depressed
bridge (Saddle nose)

- Ears:
Small, low set

- Broad, Short
Neck

- Protruding
Abdomen

- Genitalia:
Small penis
Cryptorchidism

- Mental Retardation With Developmental
Delays Of Varying Degrees

©2007 Nursing Education Consultants, Inc.

ASSESS CHANGES IN SENILE DEMENTIA

J	**J**udgment
A	**A**ffect
M	**M**emory
C	**C**ognition
O	**O**rientation

©2007 Nursing Education Consultants, Inc.

EATING DISORDERS

ANOREXIA NERVOSA

Intense fear of becoming fat.

Body image disturbance.

Weight ↓ at least 25% original body weight.

No known physical illness.

BULIMIA

Recurrent binge eating.

Awareness of abnormal eating pattern.

Fear of not being able to stop eating voluntarily.

Depressed mood following eating binges.

PICA

Persistent eating of non-nutritive

substances x's 1 month.

Infants → Paint, plaster, cloth.

Older children → Bugs, rocks, sand.

Adults → Chalk, starch, paper.

Pregnancy → Clay, dirt, laundry

detergent, baking soda.

©2007 Nursing Education Consultants, Inc.

C.J. MILLER

BIPOLAR DISORDER

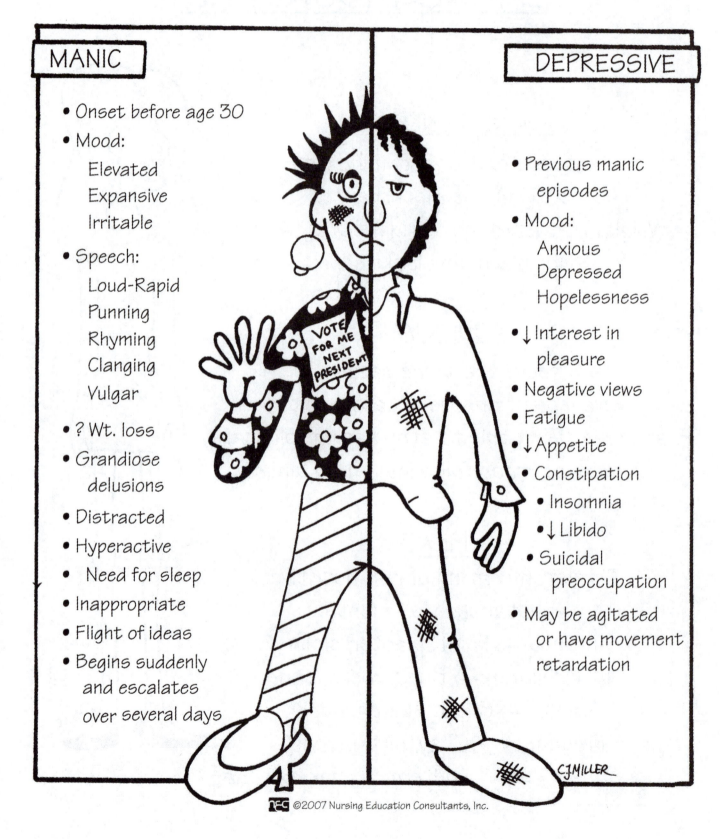

MANIC

- Onset before age 30
- Mood:
  Elevated
  Expansive
  Irritable
- Speech:
  Loud-Rapid
  Punning
  Rhyming
  Clanging
  Vulgar
- ? Wt. loss
- Grandiose delusions
- Distracted
- Hyperactive
- ↓ Need for sleep
- Inappropriate
- Flight of ideas
- Begins suddenly and escalates over several days

DEPRESSIVE

- Previous manic episodes
- Mood:
  Anxious
  Depressed
  Hopelessness
- ↓ Interest in pleasure
- Negative views
- Fatigue
- ↓ Appetite
- Constipation
- Insomnia
- ↓ Libido
- Suicidal preoccupation
- May be agitated or have movement retardation

VOTE FOR ME NEXT PRESIDENT

CJ.MILLER

©2007 Nursing Education Consultants, Inc.

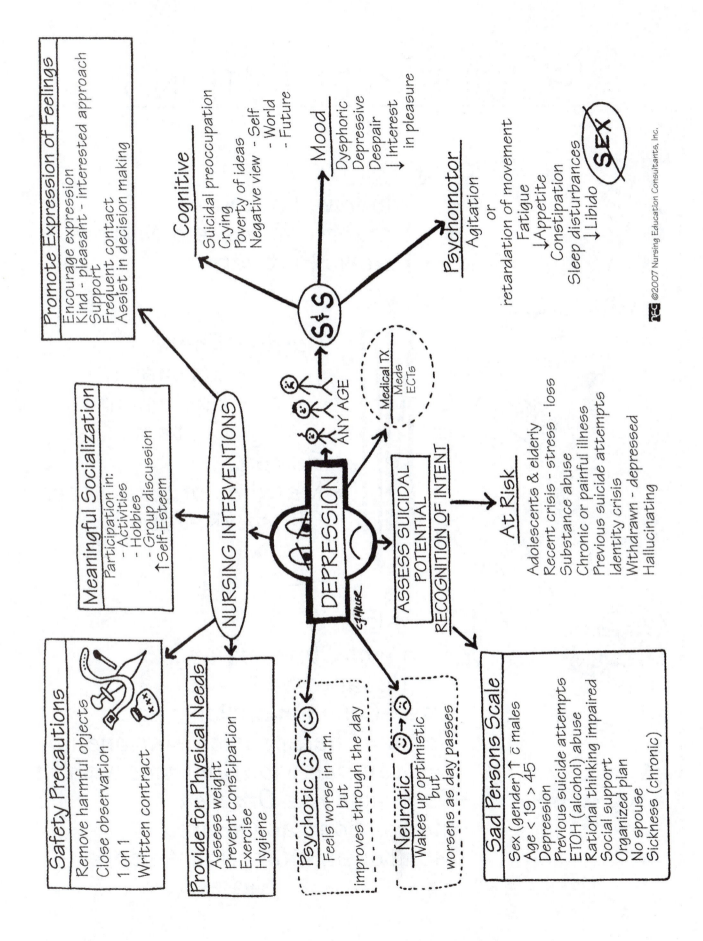

Promote Expression of Feelings
Encourage expression
Kind - pleasant - interested approach
Support
Frequent contact
Assist in decision making

Cognitive
Suicidal preoccupation
Crying
Poverty of ideas
Negative view - Self
- World
- Future

Mood
Dysphoric
Depressive
Despair
↓Interest in pleasure

Psychomotor
Agitation
or
retardation of movement
Fatigue
↓Appetite
Constipation
Sleep disturbances
↓Libido
SEX

©2007 Nursing Education Consultants, Inc.

S↓S

ANY AGE

Medical TX
Meds
ECTs

NURSING INTERVENTIONS

DEPRESSION
cjmiller

Meaningful Socialization
Participation in:
- Activities
- Hobbies
- Group discussion
↑Self-Esteem

ASSESS SUICIDAL POTENTIAL
RECOGNITION OF INTENT

At Risk
Adolescents & elderly
Recent crisis - stress - loss
Substance abuse
Chronic or painful illness
Previous suicide attempts
Identity crisis
Withdrawn - depressed
Hallucinating

Safety Precautions
Remove harmful objects
Close observation
1 on 1
Written contract

Provide for Physical Needs
Assess weight
Prevent constipation
Exercise
Hygiene

Psychotic ☹→☺
Feels worse in a.m.
but
improves through the day

Neurotic ☺→☹
Wakes up optimistic
but
worsens as day passes

Sad Persons Scale
Sex (gender) ↑ c̄ males
Age < 19 > 45
Depression
Previous suicide attempts
ETOH (alcohol) abuse
Rational thinking impaired
Social support
Organized plan
No spouse
Sickness (chronic)

SUICIDE PRECAUTIONS

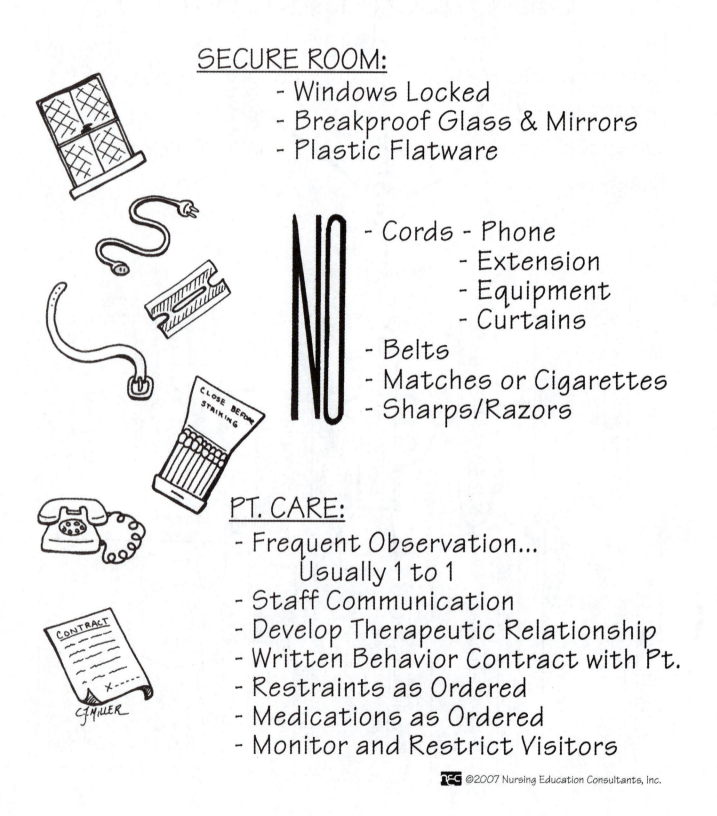

SECURE ROOM:
- Windows Locked
- Breakproof Glass & Mirrors
- Plastic Flatware

NO
- Cords - Phone
  - Extension
  - Equipment
  - Curtains
- Belts
- Matches or Cigarettes
- Sharps/Razors

PT. CARE:
- Frequent Observation...
  Usually 1 to 1
- Staff Communication
- Develop Therapeutic Relationship
- Written Behavior Contract with Pt.
- Restraints as Ordered
- Medications as Ordered
- Monitor and Restrict Visitors

SCHIZOPHRENIA

- Loss of Ego Boundaries
- Inability to Trust
- Withdrawn or Peculiar Behavior
- Indifferent - Aloof
- Love/Hate Feelings
- Personality Changes
- Confused -
    Chaotic Thoughts
- Retreat to
    Fantasy World
- Autism

- Auditory Hallucinations
    & Delusions
- Hypersensitivity to Sound,
    Sight & Smell
- Difficulty Relating to Others
- Negativism
- Religiosity
- Lack of Social Awareness
- Disorganized

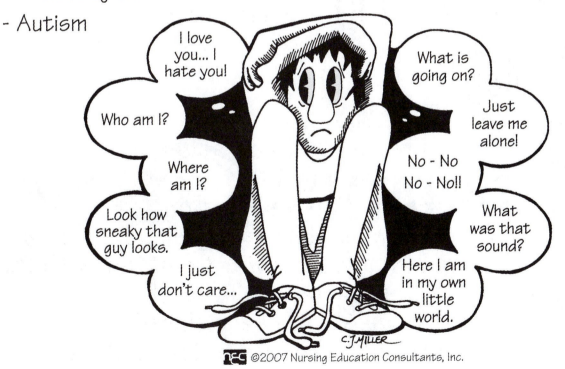

EYE MEDICATIONS

MIOTIC

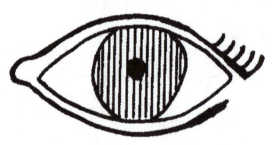

(Little Word - Little Pupil)

MYDRIATIC

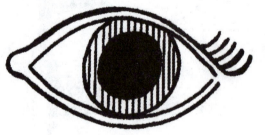

(Big Word - Big Pupil)

CATARACT

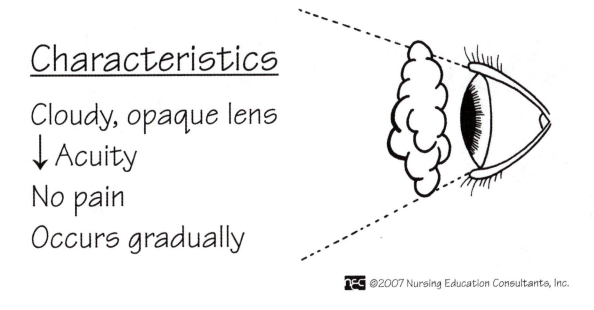

Characteristics

Cloudy, opaque lens
↓ Acuity
No pain
Occurs gradually

©2007 Nursing Education Consultants, Inc.

Treatment

Removal of lens with
lens implant

HYPERTHYROIDISM

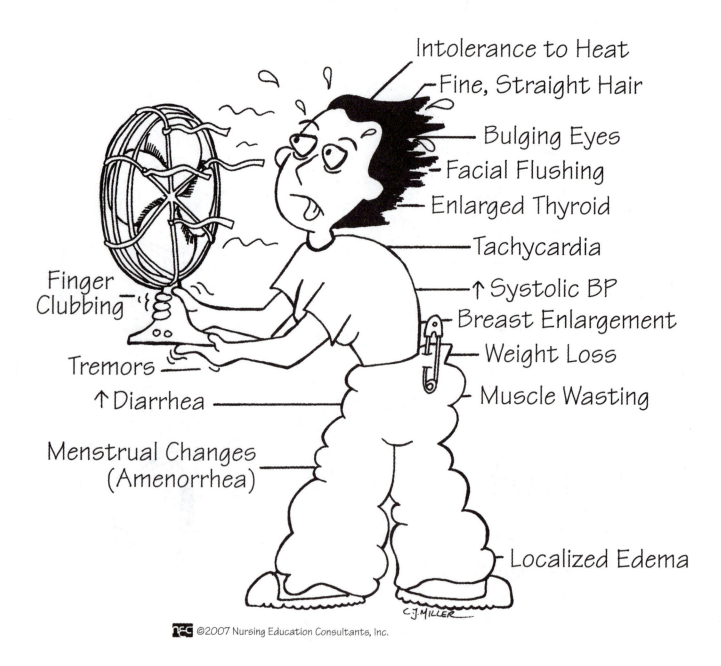

Intolerance to Heat
Fine, Straight Hair
Bulging Eyes
Facial Flushing
Enlarged Thyroid
Tachycardia
↑Systolic BP
Breast Enlargement
Weight Loss
Muscle Wasting
Localized Edema

Finger Clubbing
Tremors
↑Diarrhea
Menstrual Changes (Amenorrhea)

C.J. MILLER

HYPOTHYROIDISM

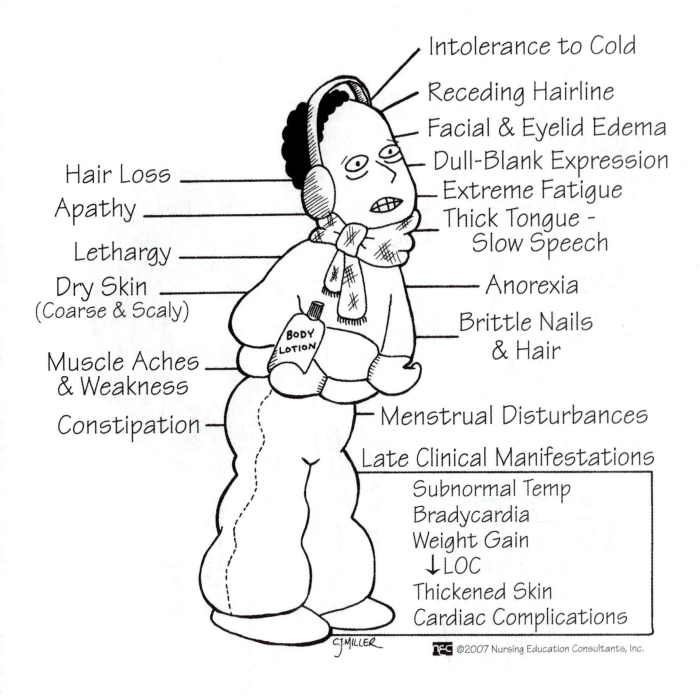

Intolerance to Cold

Receding Hairline

Facial & Eyelid Edema

Dull-Blank Expression

Extreme Fatigue

Thick Tongue - Slow Speech

Hair Loss

Apathy

Lethargy

Dry Skin (Coarse & Scaly)

Anorexia

Brittle Nails & Hair

Muscle Aches & Weakness

Constipation

Menstrual Disturbances

Late Clinical Manifestations

Subnormal Temp
Bradycardia
Weight Gain
↓LOC
Thickened Skin
Cardiac Complications

CJ.MILLER

©2007 Nursing Education Consultants, Inc.

DIABETES INSIPIDUS

History of → Head Injury or Pituitary Tumor or Craniotomy

 ©2007 Nursing Education Consultants, Inc.

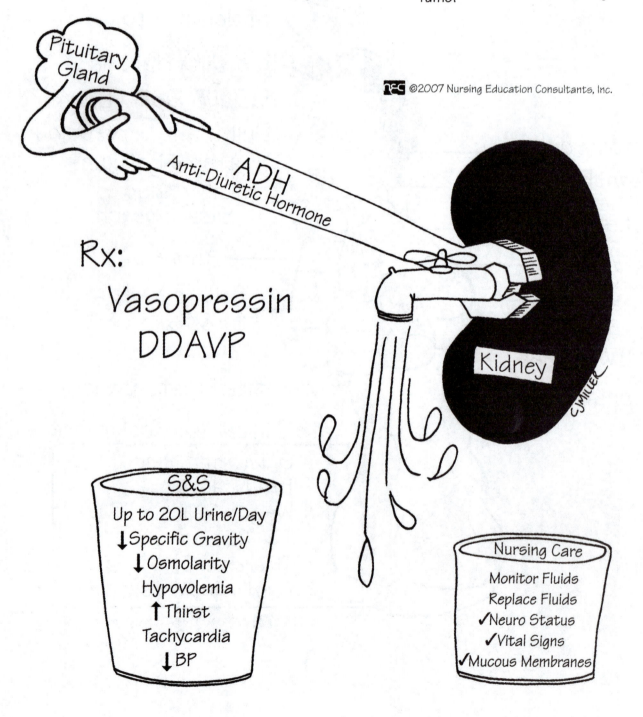

Pituitary Gland

ADH
Anti-Diuretic Hormone

Rx:

Vasopressin
DDAVP

Kidney

S&S

Up to 20L Urine/Day
↓ Specific Gravity
↓ Osmolarity
Hypovolemia
↑ Thirst
Tachycardia
↓ BP

Nursing Care

Monitor Fluids
Replace Fluids
✓ Neuro Status
✓ Vital Signs
✓ Mucous Membranes

DIABETES MELLITUS - TYPE 1
SIGNS & SYMPTOMS:

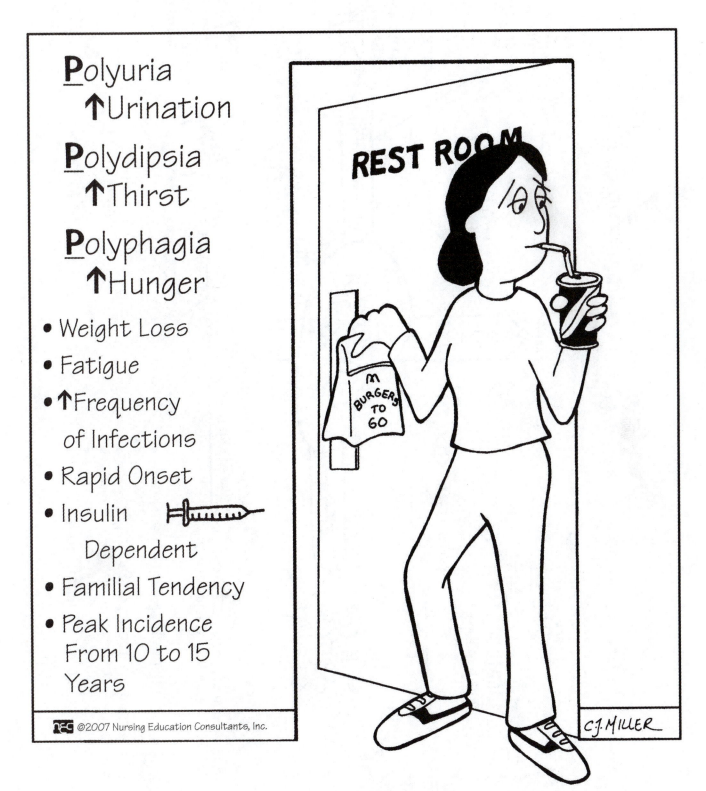

Polyuria
↑Urination

Polydipsia
↑Thirst

Polyphagia
↑Hunger

- Weight Loss
- Fatigue
- ↑Frequency
  of Infections
- Rapid Onset
- Insulin
  Dependent
- Familial Tendency
- Peak Incidence
  From 10 to 15
  Years

CJ.MILLER

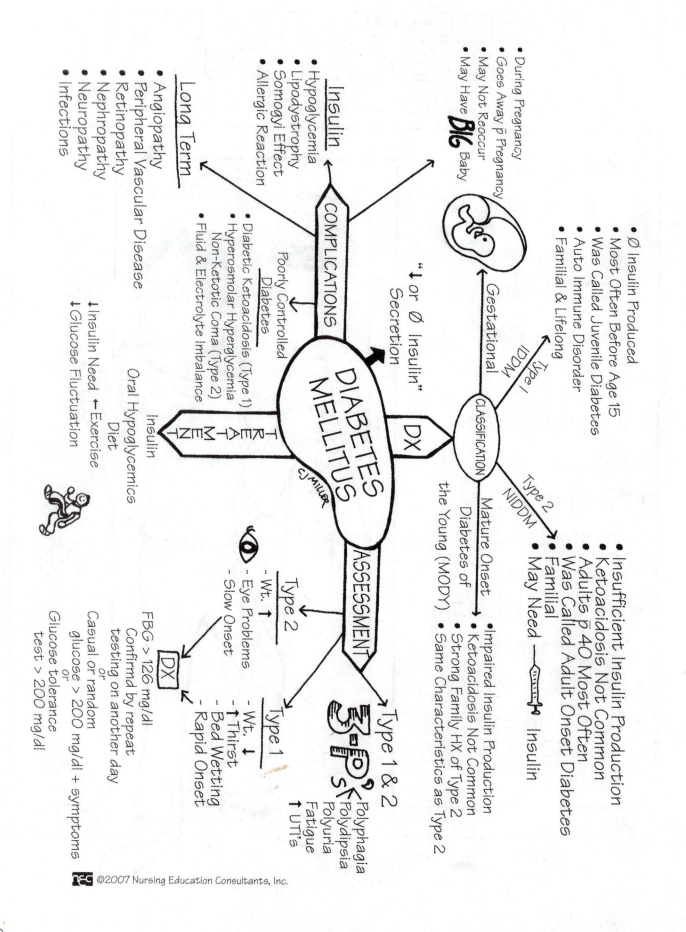

DIABETES MELLITUS

"↓ or ∅ Insulin" Secretion

COMPLICATIONS

Poorly Controlled Diabetes

- Diabetic Ketoacidosis (Type 1)
- Hyperosmolar Hyperglycemia Non-Ketotic Coma (Type 2)
- Fluid & Electrolyte Imbalance

Long Term

- Angiopathy
- Peripheral Vascular Disease
- Retinopathy
- Nephropathy
- Neuropathy
- Infections

Insulin

- Hypoglycemia
- Lipodystrophy
- Somogyi Effect
- Allergic Reaction

B₆ Baby

- During Pregnancy
- Goes Away p̄ Pregnancy
- May Not Reoccur
- May Have B₆ Baby

CLASSIFICATION

Gestational

IDDM — Type 1

- ∅ Insulin Produced
- Most Often Before Age 15
- Was Called Juvenile Diabetes
- Auto Immune Disorder
- Familial & Lifelong

NIDDM — Type 2

- Insufficient Insulin Production
- Ketoacidosis Not Common
- Adults p̄ 40 Most Often
- Was Called Adult Onset Diabetes
- Familial
- May Need — Insulin

Mature Onset Diabetes of the Young (MODY)

- Impaired Insulin Production
- Ketoacidosis Not Common
- Strong Family HX of Type 2
- Same Characteristics as Type 2

DX

Type 1 & 2

3 P's → Polyphagia
Polydipsia
Polyuria
↑ Fatigue
↑ UTI's

Type 1

- Wt. ↓
- ↑ Thirst
- Bed Wetting
- Rapid Onset

Type 2

- Wt. ↑
- Eye Problems ↑
- Slow Onset

DX

FBG > 126 mg/dl
Confirmed by repeat testing on another day
or
Casual or random glucose > 200 mg/dl + symptoms
or
Glucose tolerance test > 200 mg/dl

TREATMENT

- Insulin
- Oral Hypoglycemics
- Diet

↑ Insulin Need ← Exercise
↓ Glucose Fluctuation

ASSESSMENT

CJ MILLER

BLOOD SUGAR MNEMONIC

HOT & DRY = SUGAR HIGH

COLD & CLAMMY = NEED SOME CANDY

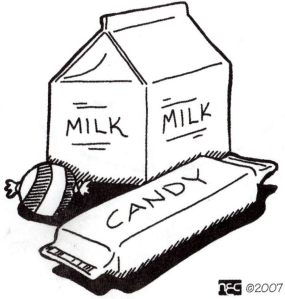

TRIANGLE OF DIABETES MANAGEMENT

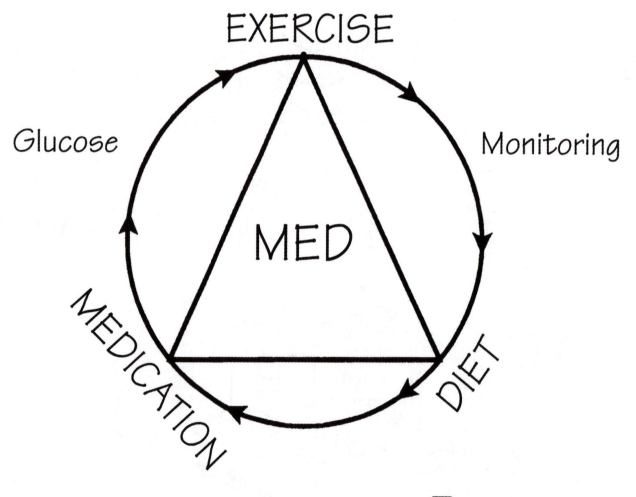

EXERCISE

Glucose

Monitoring

MED

MEDICATION

DIET

HYPOGLYCEMIA

T Tachycardia

I Irritability

R Restless

E Excessive Hunger

D Diaphoresis

Depression

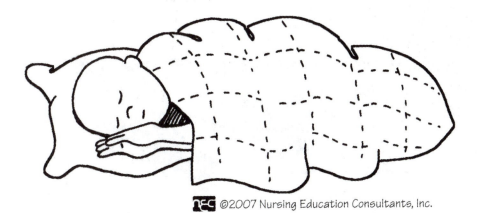

@2007 Nursing Education Consultants, Inc.

ADDISON'S DISEASE
Adrenocortical Insufficiency

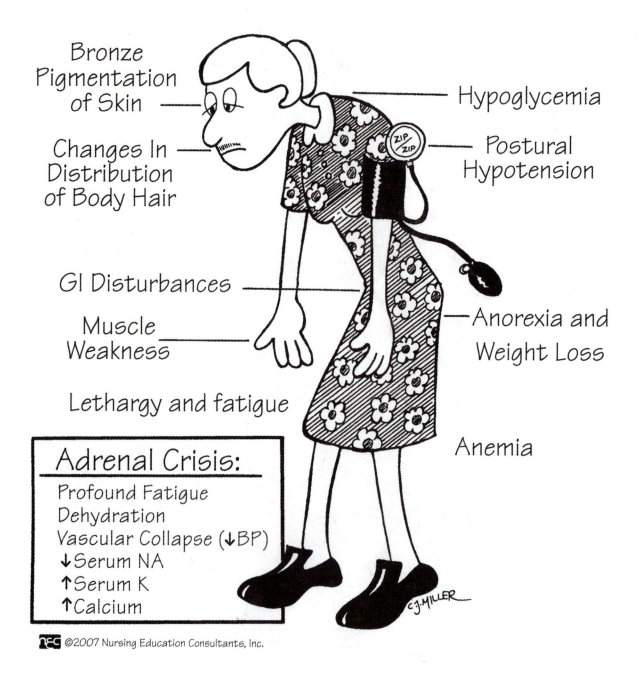

Bronze Pigmentation of Skin

Changes In Distribution of Body Hair

Hypoglycemia

Postural Hypotension

GI Disturbances

Muscle Weakness

Lethargy and fatigue

Anorexia and Weight Loss

Anemia

Adrenal Crisis:
Profound Fatigue
Dehydration
Vascular Collapse (↓BP)
↓Serum NA
↑Serum K
↑Calcium

C.J. MILLER

CUSHING'S SYNDROME

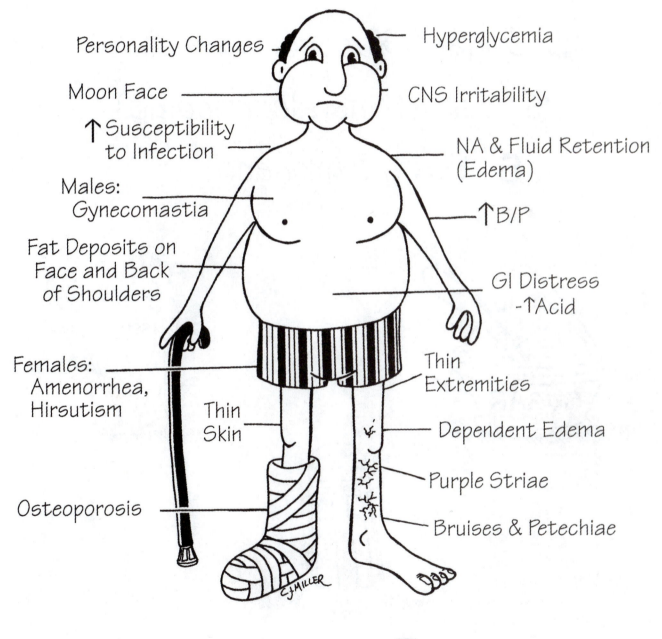

Personality Changes

Moon Face

↑ Susceptibility to Infection

Males: Gynecomastia

Fat Deposits on Face and Back of Shoulders

Females: Amenorrhea, Hirsutism

Thin Skin

Osteoporosis

Hyperglycemia

CNS Irritability

NA & Fluid Retention (Edema)

↑B/P

GI Distress -↑Acid

Thin Extremities

Dependent Edema

Purple Striae

Bruises & Petechiae

ADRENAL GLAND HORMONES

S Sugar (Glucocorticoids)

S Salt (Mineralcorticoids)

S Sex (Androgens)

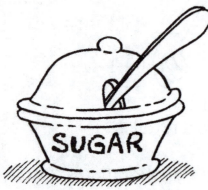

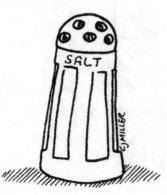

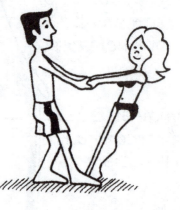

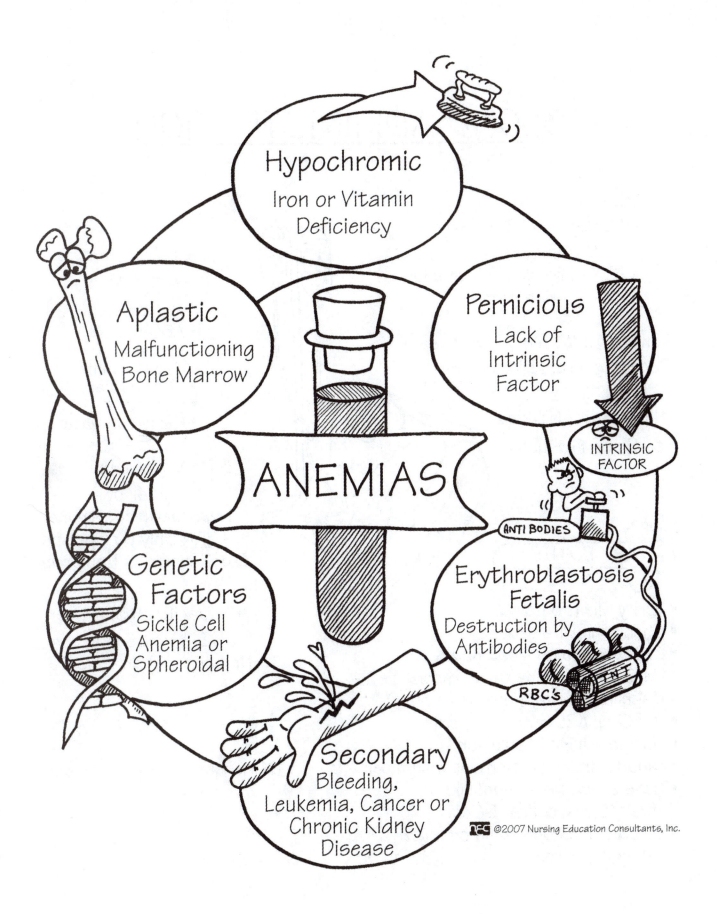

ANEMIAS

Hypochromic
Iron or Vitamin Deficiency

Aplastic
Malfunctioning Bone Marrow

Pernicious
Lack of Intrinsic Factor

INTRINSIC FACTOR

ANTIBODIES

Genetic Factors
Sickle Cell Anemia or Spheroidal

Erythroblastosis Fetalis
Destruction by Antibodies

RBC's

Secondary
Bleeding, Leukemia, Cancer or Chronic Kidney Disease

59

BLOOD ADMINISTRATION

* Determine Client's
  - Allergies
  - Previous Transfusion Reactions

* Administer Within 30 Minutes of Receiving From Blood Bank.

* Never Add ANY Meds to Blood Products.

* Check Crossmatch Record With

  2 Nurses:
  - ABO-Group
  - RH Type
  - Client's Name
  - ID Blood Band
  - Hospital #
  - Expiration Date

* Do <u>NOT</u> Warm Unless Risk of Hypothermic Response <u>THEN</u> Only By Specific Blood Warming Equipment.

* Infuse Each Unit Over 2-4 Hours <u>BUT</u> No Longer Than 4 Hours.

KEY POINTS

- Verify Client's ID
- Check the Dr's Order.
- Check labels on blood bag & blood bank transfusion record
- Baseline vitals - (Then per policy).
- #18G or #20G gauge needle.
- Normal saline IV solution.
- Blood administration set with filter.
- Severe reactions most likely first 15 min & first 50cc.
- Blood tubing should be changed after 4 hours.

©2007 Nursing Education Consultants, Inc.

BLOOD TRANSFUSION REACTION

Febrile Reaction:
- Chills • Fever • Headache
- Flushing • Tachycardia • ↑Anxiety

Allergic Reaction:
Mild:
- Hives • Pruritus
- Facial Flushing

Severe:
- Severe Shortness of Breath
- Bronchospasm
- Anxiety

Hemolytic Transfusion Reaction:
- Low Back Pain
- Hypotension
- Tachycardia
- Fever and Chills
- Chest Pain
- Tachypnea
- Hemoglobinuria
- May Have Immediate Onset

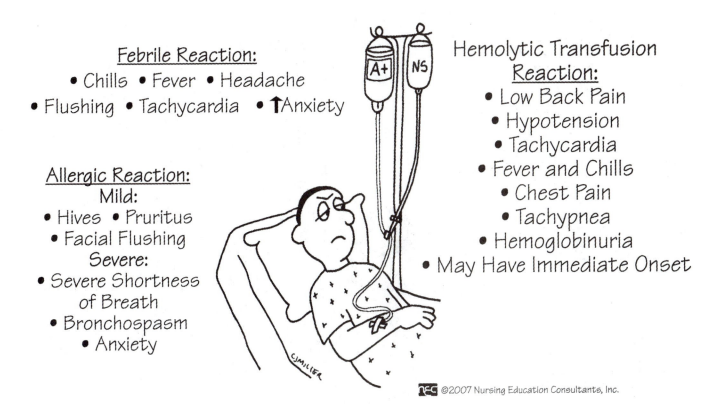

@2007 Nursing Education Consultants, Inc.

⭐ **Nursing Implications:**
- Stop Transfusion and notify Physician.
- Change IV Tubing.
- Treat symptoms if present → O2, fluids, epinephrine as ordered.
- Recheck crossmatch record with unit.

HEMOLYTIC REACTIONS
- Obtain 2 blood samples distal to infusion site.
- Obtain first UA-test for hemoglobinuria.
- Monitor fluid/electrolyte balance.
- Evaluate serum calcium levels.

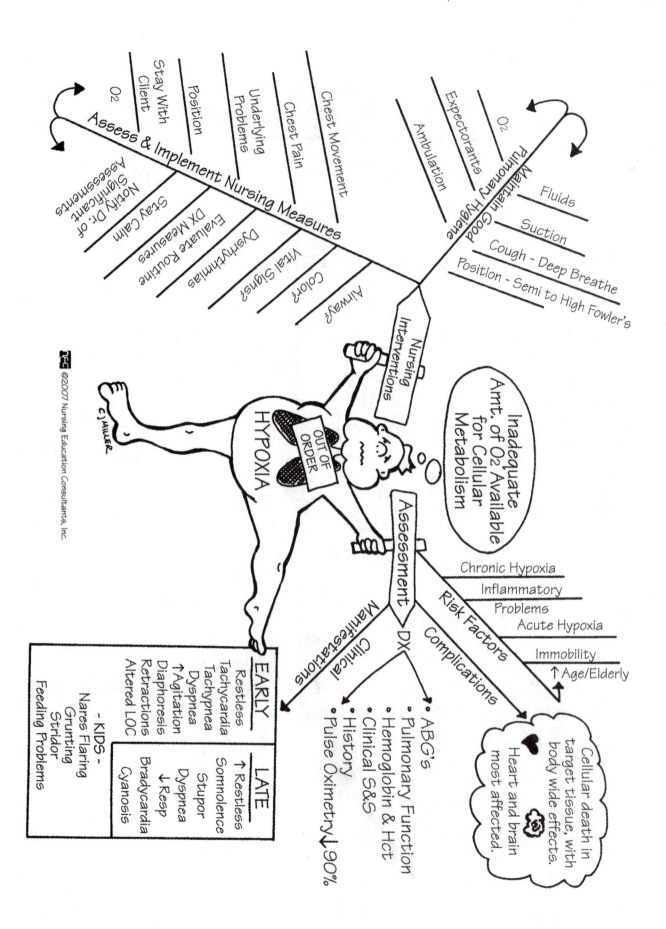

HYPOXIA

OUT OF ORDER

Inadequate Amt. of O_2 Available for Cellular Metabolism

Assess & Implement Nursing Measures

- Assess
  - Airway?
  - Color?
  - Vital Signs?
  - Dysrhythmias
  - Evaluate Routine DX Measures
  - Stay Calm
  - Notify Dr. of Significant Assessments
- Implement
  - Chest Movement
  - Chest Pain
  - Underlying Problems
  - Position
  - Stay With Client
  - O_2

Maintain Good Pulmonary Hygiene
- O_2
- Expectorants
- Ambulation
- Fluids
- Suction
- Cough - Deep Breathe
- Position - Semi to High Fowler's

Nursing Interventions

Assessment

Manifestations — Clinical

EARLY	LATE
Restless	↑ Restless
Tachycardia	Somnolence
Tachypnea	Stupor
Dyspnea	Dyspnea
↑Agitation	↓ Resp
Diaphoresis	Bradycardia
Retractions	Cyanosis
Altered LOC	

- KIDS -
- Nares Flaring
- Grunting
- Stridor
- Feeding Problems

DX
- ABG's
- Pulmonary Function
- Hemoglobin & Hct
- Clinical S&S
- History
- Pulse Oximetry ↓90%

Risk Factors
- Chronic Hypoxia
- Inflammatory Problems
- Acute Hypoxia
- Immobility
- ↑ Age/Elderly

Complications
Cellular death in target tissue, with body wide effects. Heart and brain most affected.

©2007 Nursing Education Consultants, Inc.

C.J. MILLER

COPD

CHRONIC AIRFLOW LIMITATION
"EMPHYSEMA AND CHRONIC BRONCHITIS"

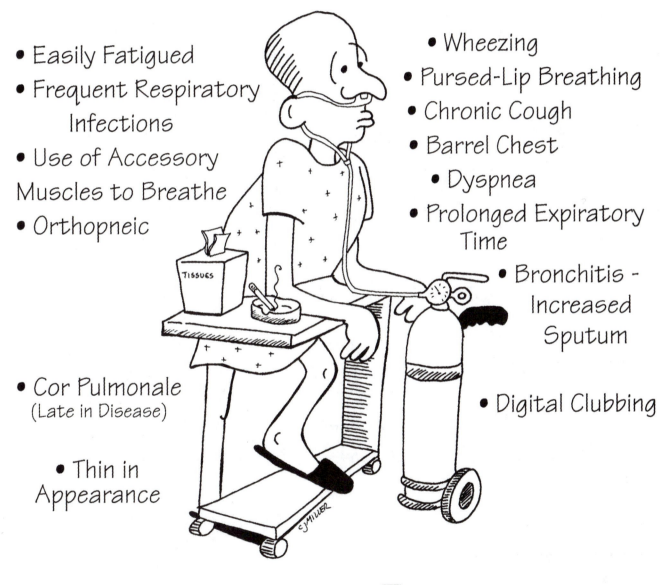

- Easily Fatigued
- Frequent Respiratory Infections
- Use of Accessory Muscles to Breathe
- Orthopneic

- Cor Pulmonale (Late in Disease)

- Thin in Appearance

- Wheezing
- Pursed-Lip Breathing
- Chronic Cough
- Barrel Chest
- Dyspnea
- Prolonged Expiratory Time
- Bronchitis - Increased Sputum
- Digital Clubbing

EMPHYSEMA
"PINK PUFFER"

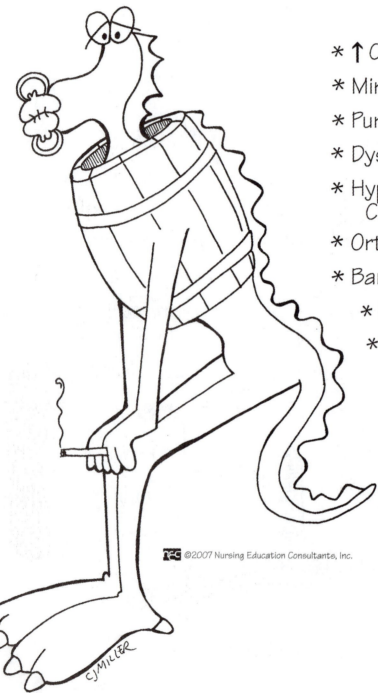

* ↑ CO_2 Retention (Pink)
* Minimal Cyanosis
* Purse Lip Breathing
* Dyspnea
* Hyperresonance on Chest Percussion
* Orthopneic
* Barrel Chest
* Exertional Dyspnea
* Prolonged Expiratory Time
* Speaks in Short Jerky Sentences
* Anxious
* Use of Accessory Muscles to Breathe
* Thin Appearance

CJMILLER

CHRONIC BRONCHITIS
"BLUE BLOATER"

* Color Dusky to Cyanotic
* Recurrent Cough & ↑ Sputum Production
* Hypoxia
* Hypercapnia (↑ pCO_2)
* Respiratory Acidosis
* ↑ Hbg
* ↑ Resp Rate
* Exertional Dyspnea
* ↑ Incidence in Heavy Cigarette Smokers
* Digital Clubbing

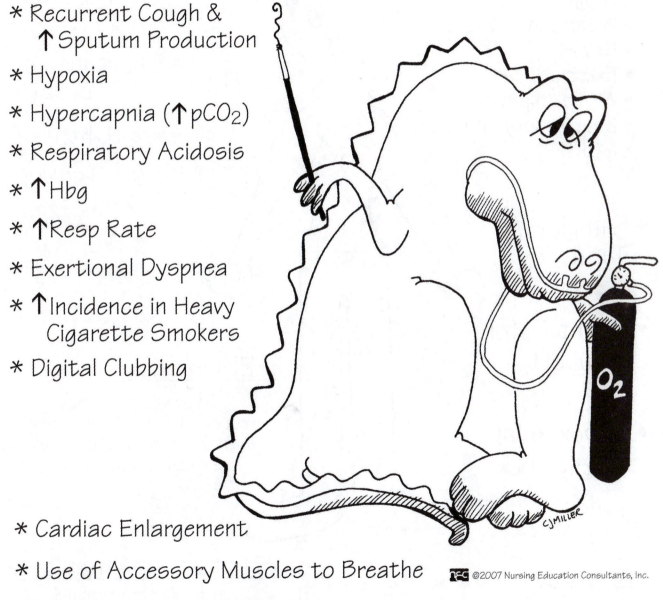

* Cardiac Enlargement
* Use of Accessory Muscles to Breathe
* Leads to Right-Sided Failure

ASTHMA
(Reactive Airway Disease)

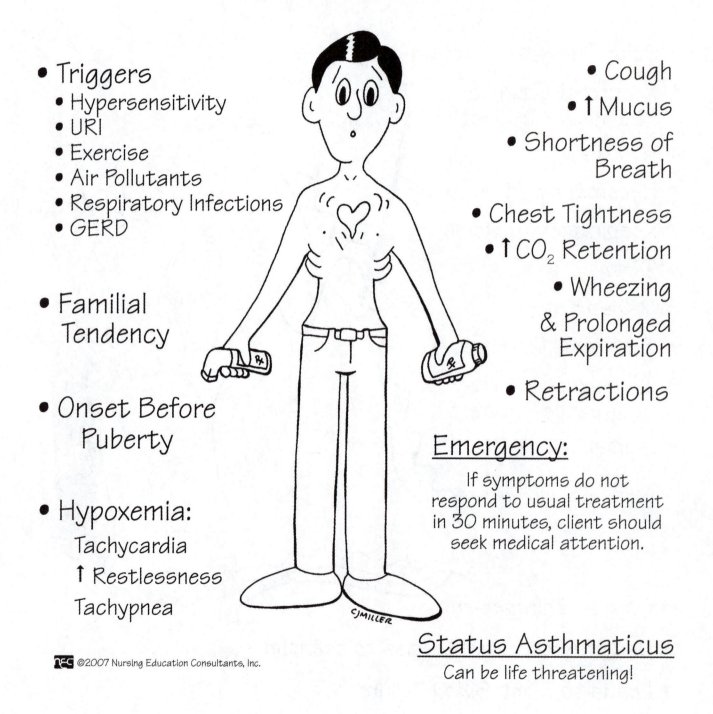

- Triggers
  - Hypersensitivity
  - URI
  - Exercise
  - Air Pollutants
  - Respiratory Infections
  - GERD

- Familial Tendency

- Onset Before Puberty

- Hypoxemia:
  - Tachycardia
  - ↑ Restlessness
  - Tachypnea

- Cough
- ↑ Mucus
- Shortness of Breath
- Chest Tightness
- ↑ CO_2 Retention
- Wheezing & Prolonged Expiration
- Retractions

Emergency:
If symptoms do not respond to usual treatment in 30 minutes, client should seek medical attention.

Status Asthmaticus
Can be life threatening!

CJMILLER

ACUTE LARYNGOTRACHEOBRONCHITIS
LTB (Croup)

- Slow Onset
- Barking Cough
- "Crowing Sounds"

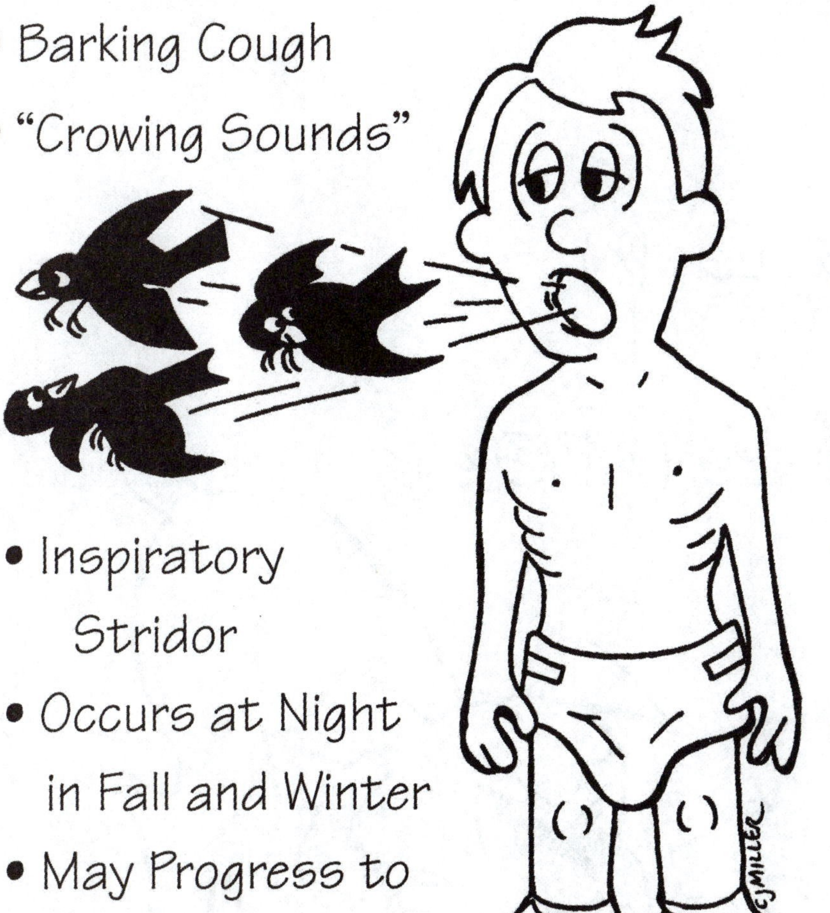

- Inspiratory Stridor
- Occurs at Night in Fall and Winter
- May Progress to Hypoxic State
- May Have Slight Temperature (<102°)

- Commonly Occurs Age 3 Months to 3 Years
- U.R.I.'s Frequently Precede LTB
- Restlessness
- Supra-sternal Retractions
- ↑Respiratory Rate

©2007 Nursing Education Consultants, Inc.

PULMONARY EDEMA

M
A
D

Meds → Nipride, Morphine

Airway

Digitalis

D
O
G

Diuretics (Lasix)

Oxygen

Blood Gases (ABG's)

©2007 Nursing Education Consultants, Inc.

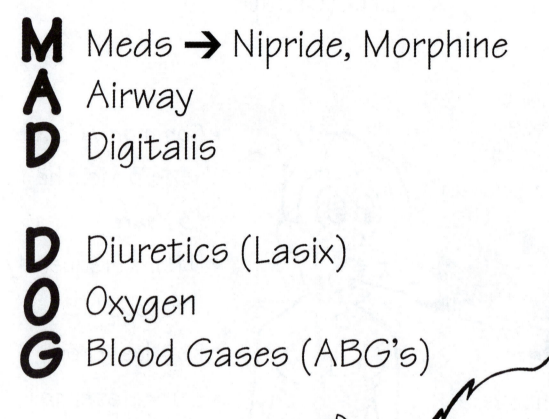

TUBERCULOSIS (TB)

- Progressive Fatigue
- Malaise
- Anorexia
- Wt. Loss

- Chronic Cough
  (Productive)

- Night Sweats
- Hemoptysis
  (Advanced State)

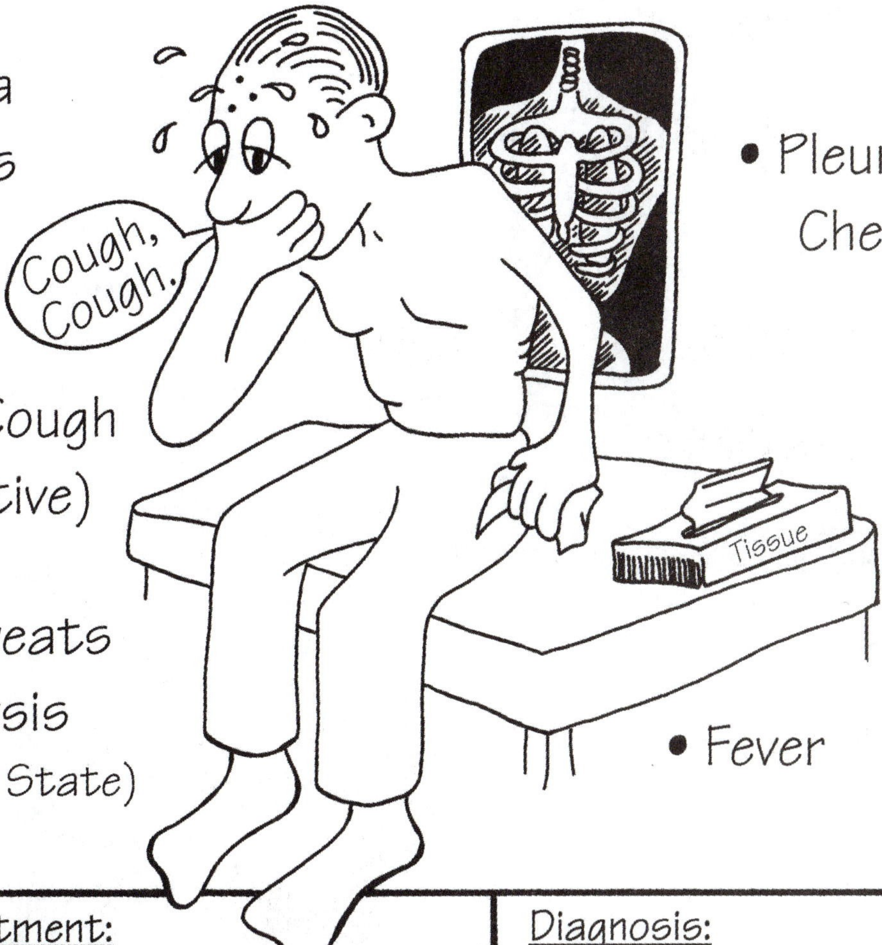

Cough, Cough.

- Pleuritic
  Chest Pain

Tissue

- Fever

Treatment:	Diagnosis:
TB Medications 6 to 12 Months	TB Skin Test (screening)
Decreased Activity	Chest X-Ray
Resp Isolation Until Negative Sputum	Sputum Studies
Frequently Out-PT Basis	(3 specimens collected
	on different days)

@2007 Nursing Education Consultants, Inc.

Sleep Apnea

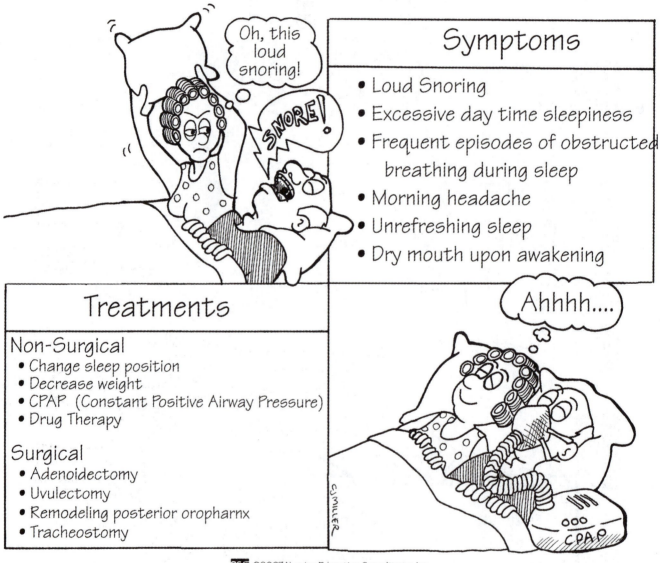

Symptoms

- Loud Snoring
- Excessive day time sleepiness
- Frequent episodes of obstructed breathing during sleep
- Morning headache
- Unrefreshing sleep
- Dry mouth upon awakening

Treatments

Non-Surgical
- Change sleep position
- Decrease weight
- CPAP (Constant Positive Airway Pressure)
- Drug Therapy

Surgical
- Adenoidectomy
- Uvulectomy
- Remodeling posterior oropharnx
- Tracheostomy

NEUROVASCULAR ASSESSMENT

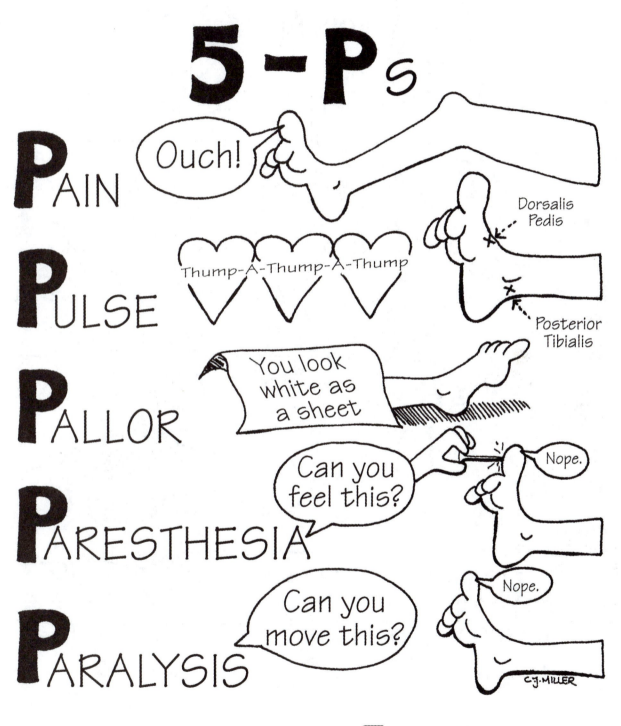

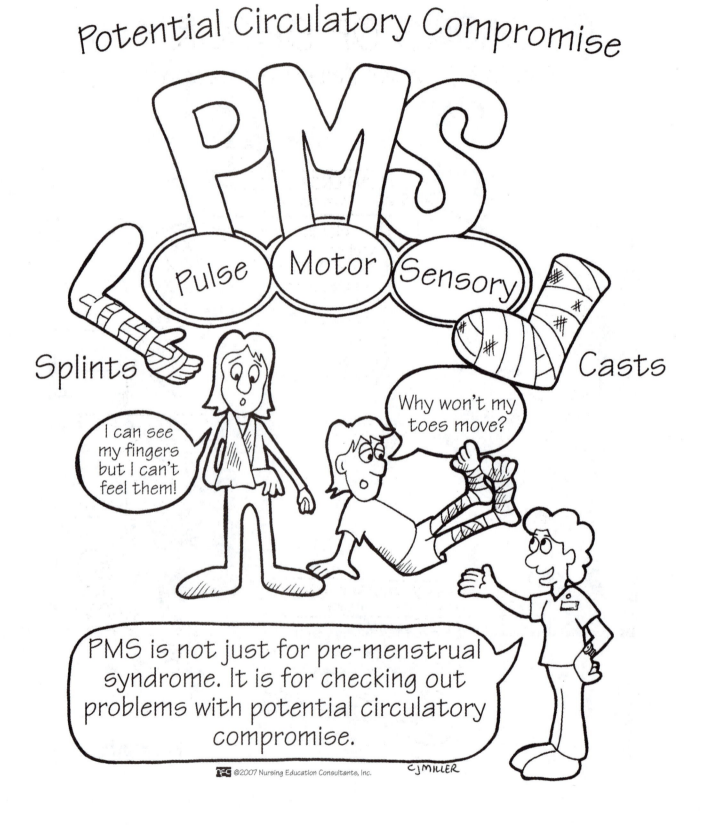

SIGNS OF SHOCK
↓ In MAP (Mean Arterial Pressure)

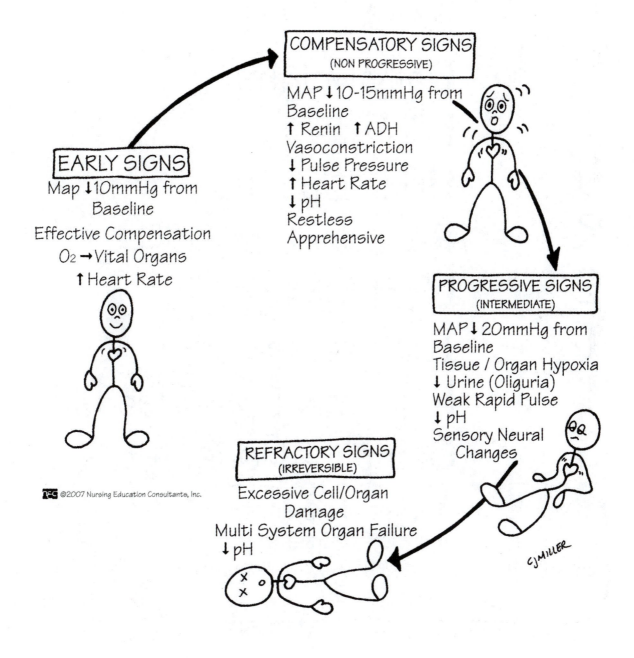

COMPENSATORY SIGNS
(NON PROGRESSIVE)

MAP ↓10-15mmHg from
Baseline
↑ Renin ↑ ADH
Vasoconstriction
↓ Pulse Pressure
↑ Heart Rate
↓ pH
Restless
Apprehensive

EARLY SIGNS

Map ↓10mmHg from
Baseline

Effective Compensation
O_2 → Vital Organs
↑ Heart Rate

PROGRESSIVE SIGNS
(INTERMEDIATE)

MAP ↓20mmHg from
Baseline
Tissue / Organ Hypoxia
↓ Urine (Oliguria)
Weak Rapid Pulse
↓ pH
Sensory Neural
Changes

REFRACTORY SIGNS
(IRREVERSIBLE)

Excessive Cell/Organ
Damage
Multi System Organ Failure
↓ pH

CJMILLER

HYPERTENSION NURSING CARE

D	**D**aily weight
I	**I** & O
U	**U**rine Output
R	**R**esponse of B/P
E	**E**lectrolytes
T	**T**ake Pulses
I	**I**schemic Episodes (TIA)
C	**C**omplications: 4 C's

- CAD
- CRF
- CHF
- CVA

COMPLICATIONS OF TRAUMA CLIENT

T Tissue Perfusion Problems

R Respiratory Problems

A Anxiety

U Unstable Clotting Factors

M Malnutrition (Fluids & Food)

A Altered Body Image

T Thromboembolism

I Infection

C Coping Problems

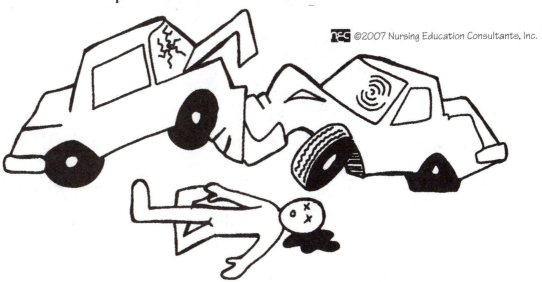

©2007 Nursing Education Consultants, Inc.

AUSCULATING HEART SOUNDS

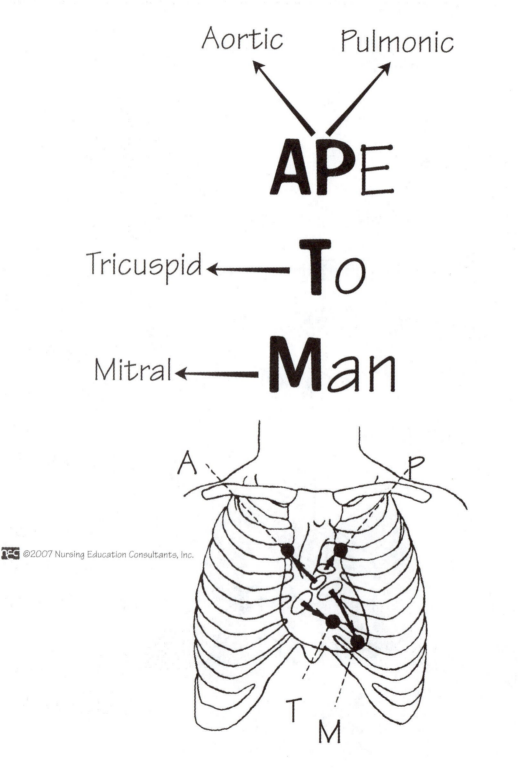

Aortic   Pulmonic

APE

Tricuspid ← To

Mitral ← Man

PRELOAD AND AFTERLOAD

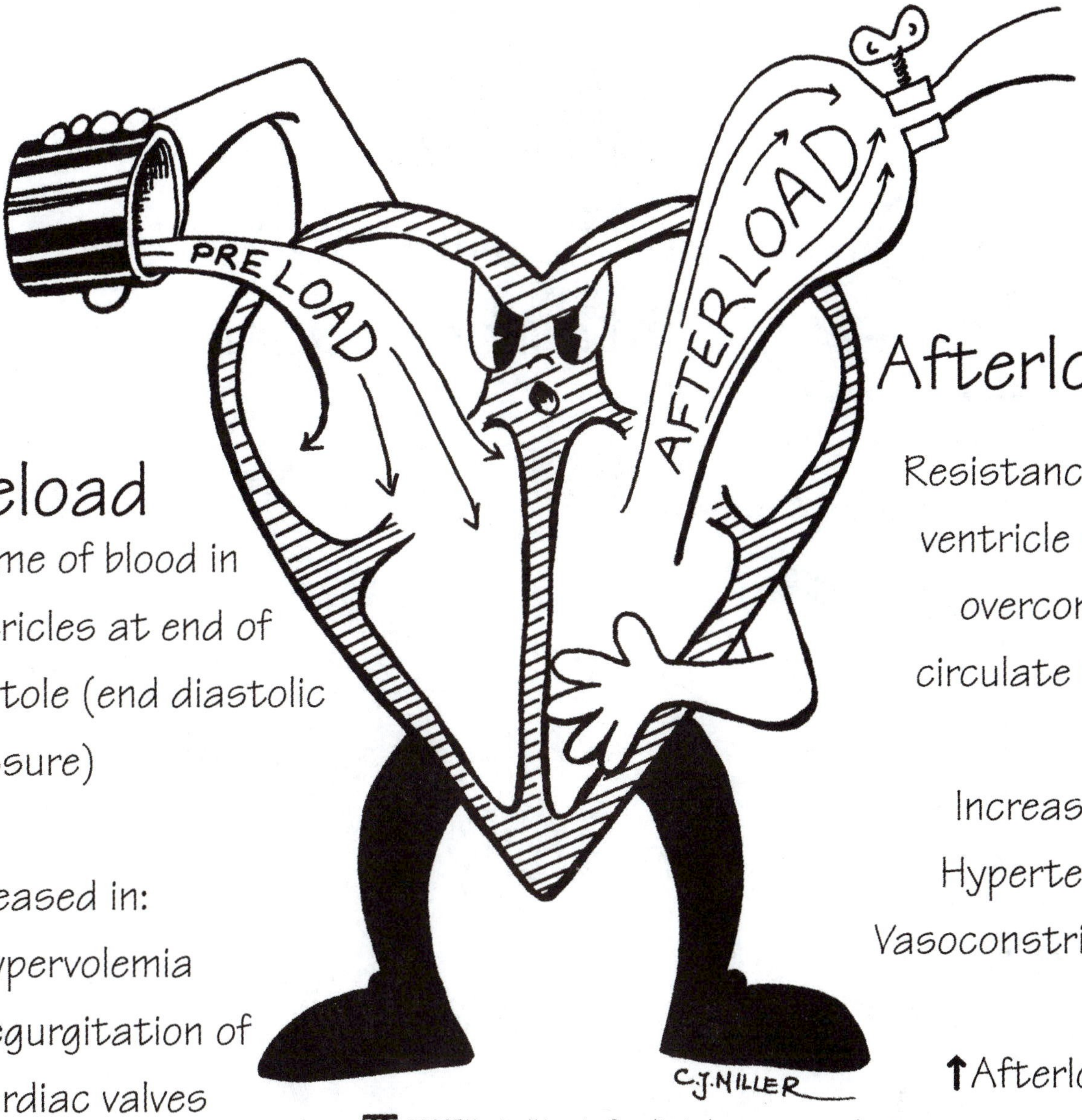

Preload
Volume of blood in ventricles at end of diastole (end diastolic pressure)

Increased in:
Hypervolemia
Regurgitation of cardiac valves
Heart Failure

Afterload
Resistance left ventricle must overcome to circulate blood

Increased in:
Hypertension
Vasoconstriction

↑Afterload =
↑ Cardiac workload

C.J.MILLER

LDL/HDL

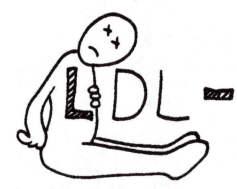

Low Density Liproprotein

Want <u>LOW</u> (↓130mg/dl) or it will lower you into the ground.

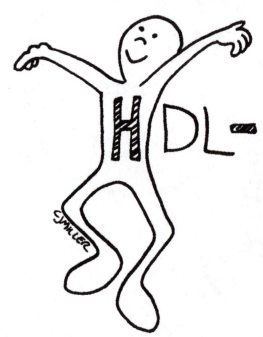

High Density Liproprotein

Want <u>HIGH</u> (↑45mg/dl) for client to feel healthy.

- MYOCARDIAL INFARCTION (MI) -
- CORONARY OCCLUSION -
- HEART ATTACK -

- Pain:
    - Sudden Onset
    - Substernal
    - Crushing
    - Tightness
    - Severe
    - Unrelieved by Nitro
    - May Radiate To: Back
        - Neck
        - Jaw
        - Shoulder
        - Arm

- Dyspnea
- Syncope (↓BP)
- Nausea
- Vomiting
- Extreme Weakness
- Diaphoresis
- Denial is Common
- ↑HR

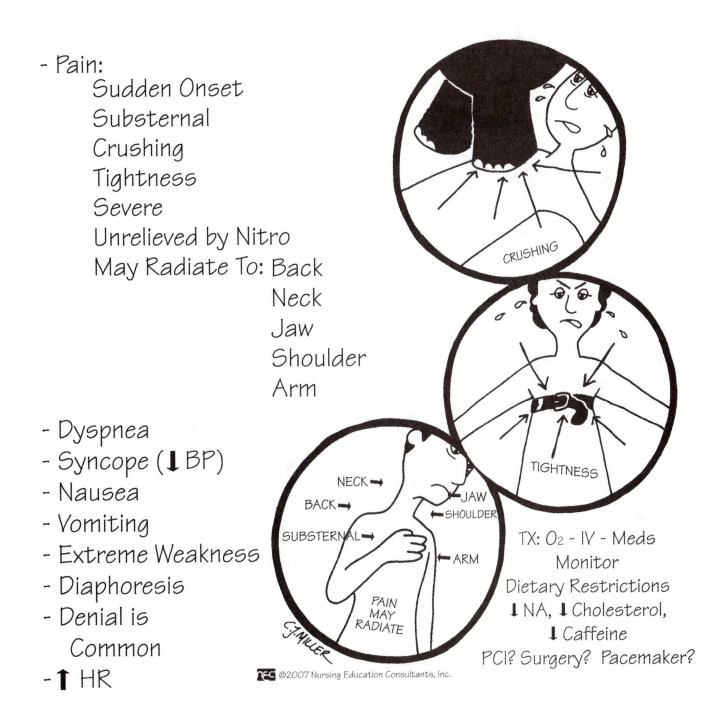

CRUSHING

TIGHTNESS

NECK →
BACK →
SUBSTERNAL →
JAW
SHOULDER
ARM
PAIN MAY RADIATE

C.J.MILLER

TX: O₂ - IV - Meds
Monitor
Dietary Restrictions
↓NA, ↓Cholesterol,
↓Caffeine
PCI? Surgery? Pacemaker?

LEFT SIDED ♥ FAILURE

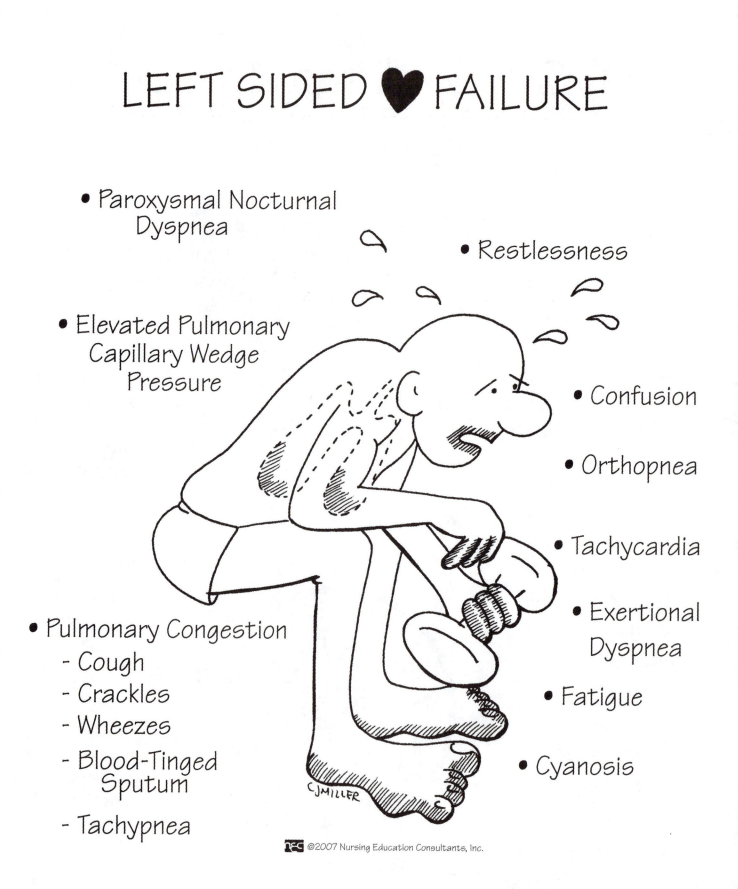

- Paroxysmal Nocturnal Dyspnea

- Restlessness

- Elevated Pulmonary Capillary Wedge Pressure

- Confusion

- Orthopnea

- Tachycardia

- Exertional Dyspnea

- Pulmonary Congestion
  - Cough
  - Crackles
  - Wheezes
  - Blood-Tinged Sputum
  - Tachypnea

- Fatigue

- Cyanosis

CJMILLER

RIGHT SIDED ♥ FAILURE
(Cor Pulmonale)

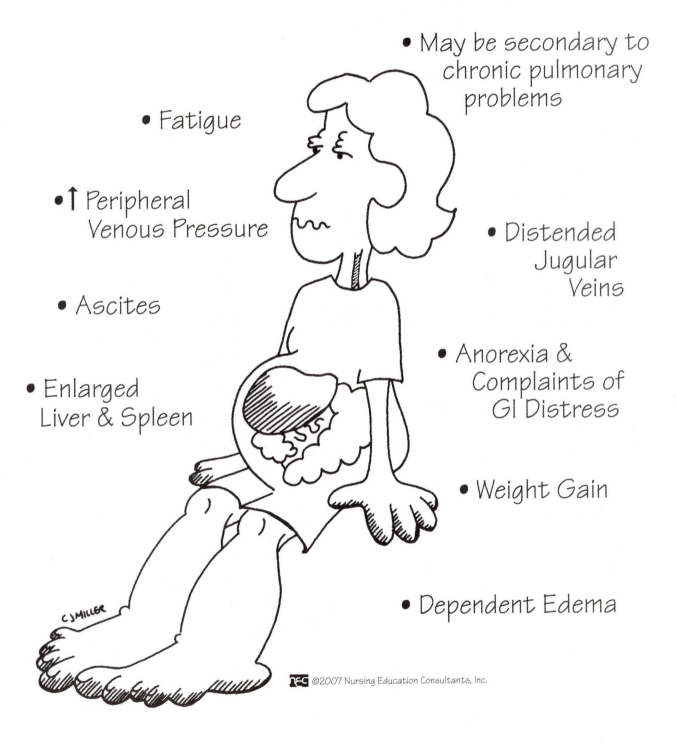

- Fatigue

- ↑ Peripheral Venous Pressure

- Ascites

- Enlarged Liver & Spleen

- May be secondary to chronic pulmonary problems

- Distended Jugular Veins

- Anorexia & Complaints of GI Distress

- Weight Gain

- Dependent Edema

CJMILLER

Cyanotic Congenital ♥ Defects

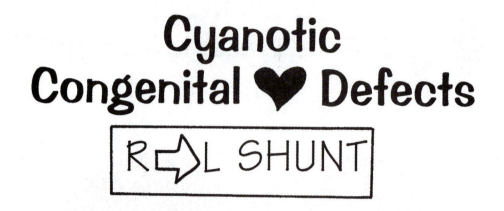

R ⇨ L SHUNT

Example:
Tetralogy of Fallot

- Squatting
- Cyanosis
- Clubbing
- Syncope

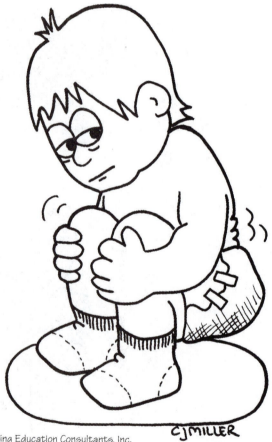

CJMILLER

CYANOTIC DEFECTS MNEMONIC

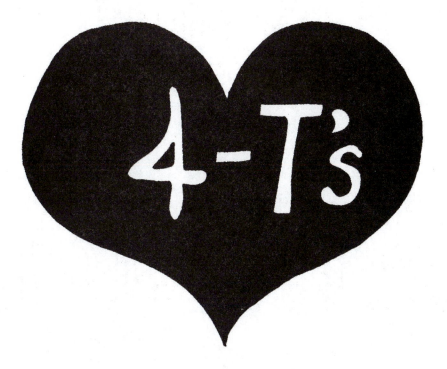

4-T's

- **T**etralogy of Fallot
- **T**runcus Arteriosus
- **T**ransposition of The Great Vessels
- **T**ricuspid Atresia

©2007 Nursing Education Consultants, Inc.

ACYANOTIC CONGENITAL 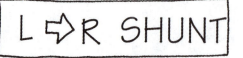 DEFECTS

L ⇨ R SHUNT

Example:
Patent Ductus Arteriosus
(PDA)
Atrial Septal Defect
(ASD)
Ventricular Septal Defect
(VSD)

- ↑ Fatigue
- ♡ Murmur
- ↑ Risk Endocarditis
- CHF
- Growth Retardation

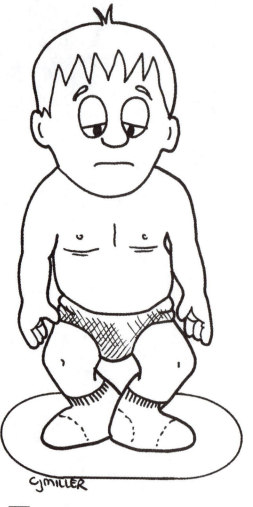

CJMILLER

CONGENITAL ♥ DEFECT SYMPTOMS

- ♥ ↑ Pulse
- ♥ ↑ Respirations
- ♥ Retarded Growth
- ♥ Dyspnea, Orthopnea
- ♥ Fatigue
- ♥ URI

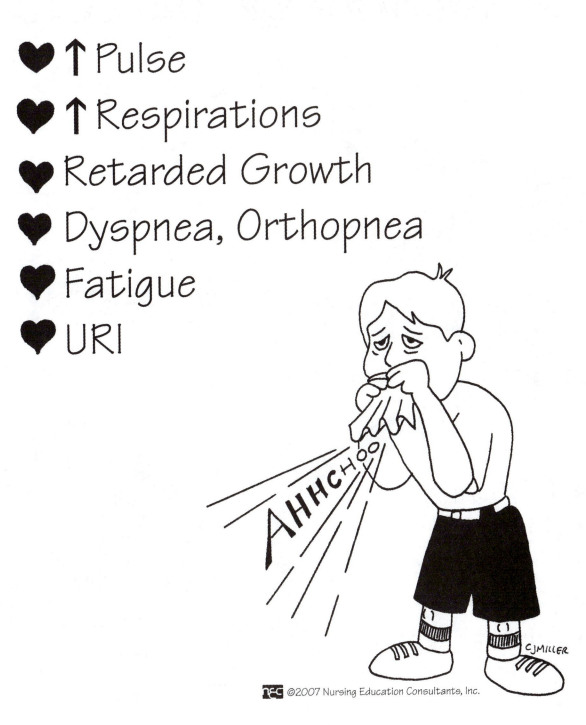

AHHCHOO

CJMILLER

nEC ©2007 Nursing Education Consultants, Inc.

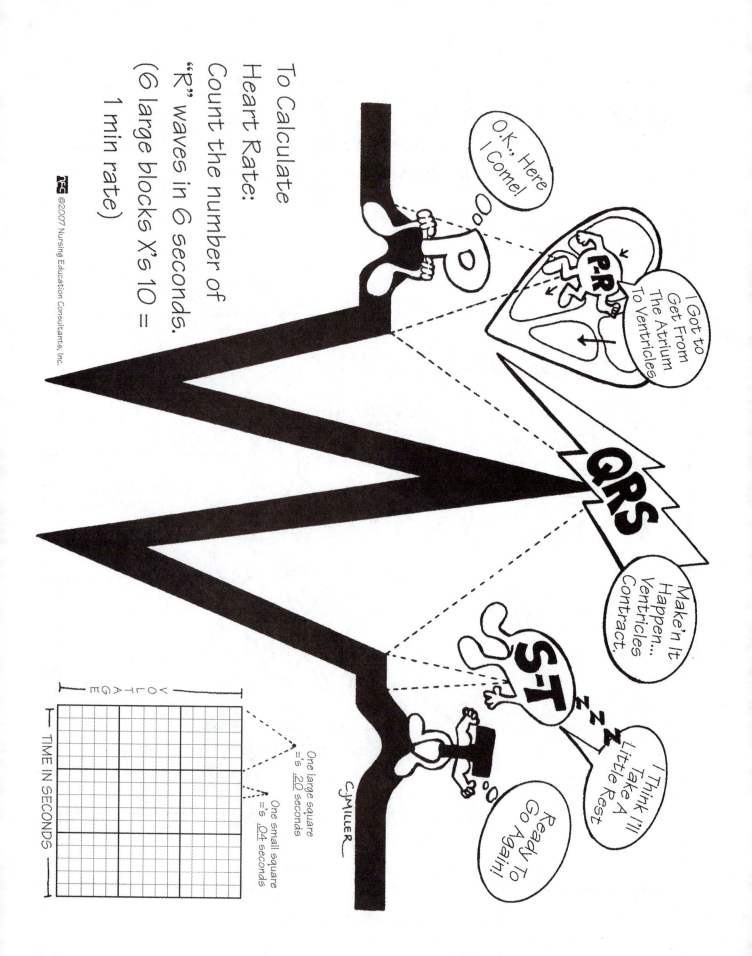

To Calculate
Heart Rate:
Count the number of
"R" waves in 6 seconds.
(6 large blocks X's 10 =
1 min rate)

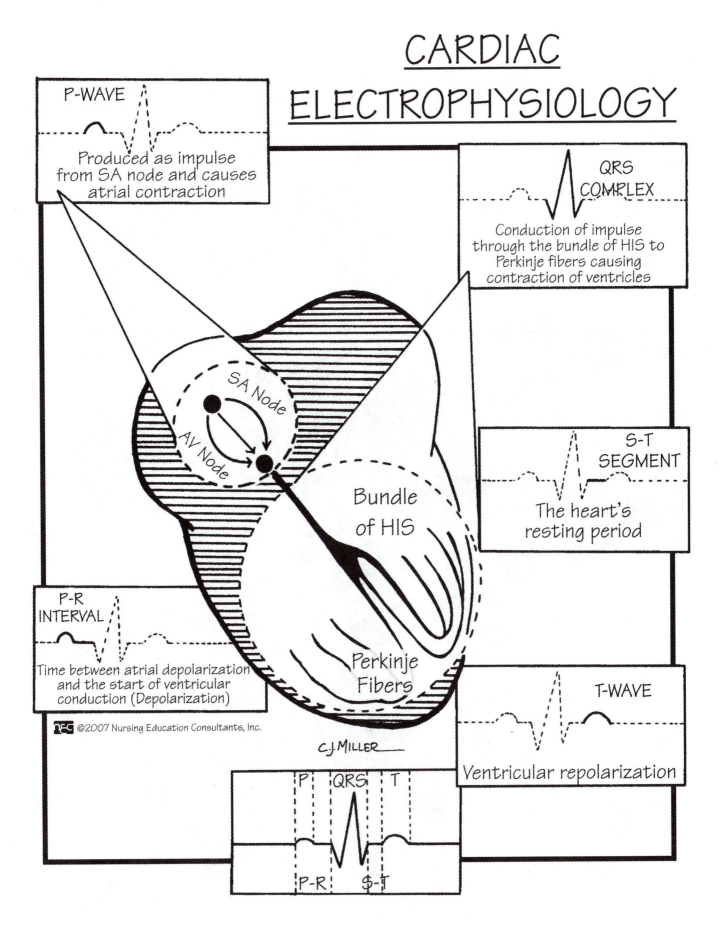

CARDIAC ELECTROPHYSIOLOGY

P-WAVE

Produced as impulse from SA node and causes atrial contraction

QRS COMPLEX

Conduction of impulse through the bundle of HIS to Perkinje fibers causing contraction of ventricles

S-T SEGMENT

The heart's resting period

P-R INTERVAL

Time between atrial depolarization and the start of ventricular conduction (Depolarization)

T-WAVE

Ventricular repolarization

SA Node

AV Node

Bundle of HIS

Perkinje Fibers

©2007 Nursing Education Consultants, Inc.

C.J. MILLER

P   QRS   T

P-R   S-T

87

PEPTIC ULCER DISEASE (PUD)

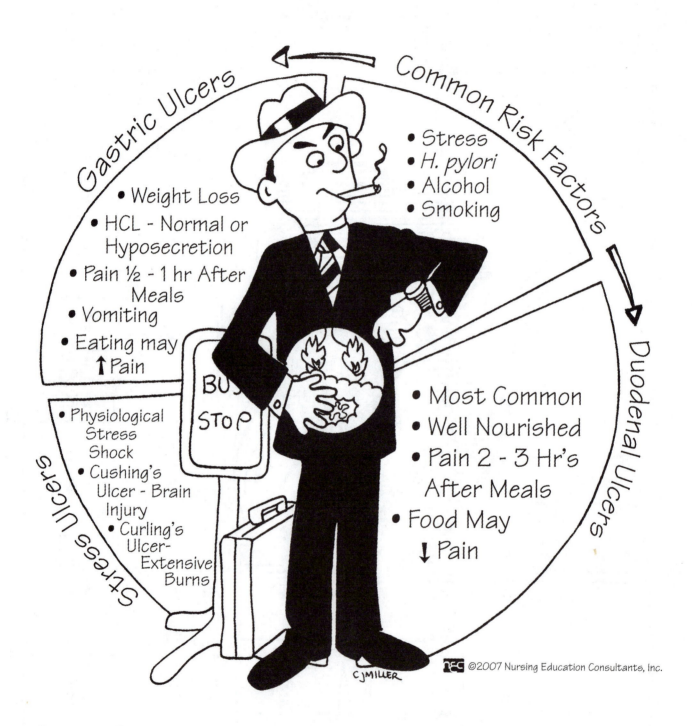

Gastric Ulcers
- Weight Loss
- HCL - Normal or Hyposecretion
- Pain ½ - 1 hr After Meals
- Vomiting
- Eating may ↑ Pain

Common Risk Factors
- Stress
- *H. pylori*
- Alcohol
- Smoking

Stress Ulcers
- Physiological Stress Shock
- Cushing's Ulcer - Brain Injury
- Curling's Ulcer- Extensive Burns

Duodenal Ulcers
- Most Common
- Well Nourished
- Pain 2 - 3 Hr's After Meals
- Food May ↓ Pain

BUS STOP

CJMILLER

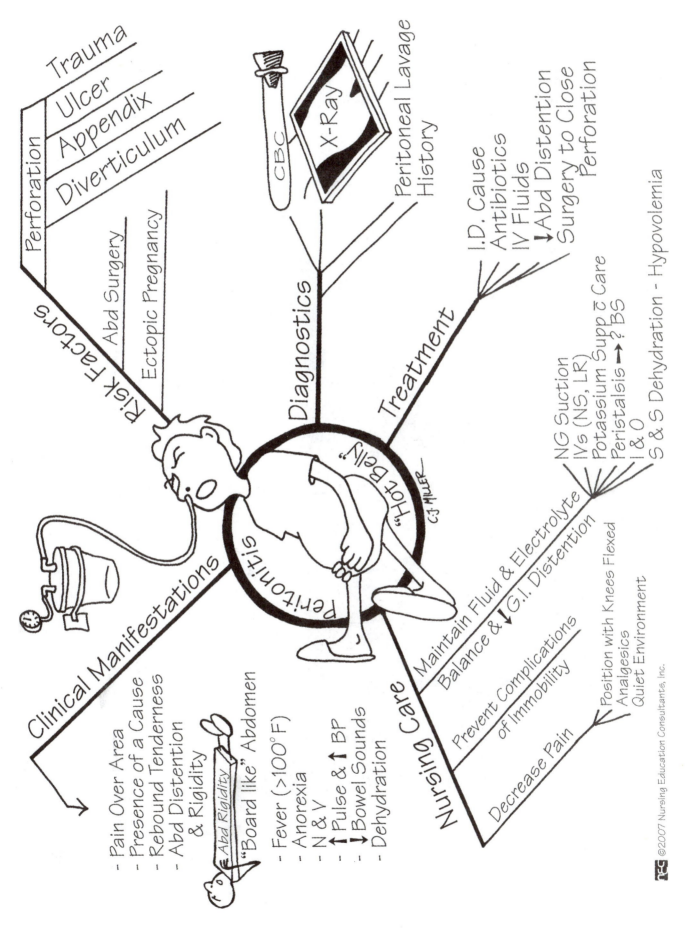

Peritonitis — "Hot Belly"

Risk Factors
- Perforation
  - Trauma
  - Ulcer
  - Appendix
  - Diverticulum
- Abd Surgery
- Ectopic Pregnancy

Diagnostics
- CBC
- X-Ray
- Peritoneal Lavage
- History

Treatment
- I.D. Cause
- Antibiotics
- IV Fluids
- ↓ Abd Distention
- Surgery to Close Perforation

Clinical Manifestations
- Pain Over Area
- Presence of a Cause
- Rebound Tenderness
- Abd Distention & Rigidity

"Board like" Abdomen — Abd Rigidity

- Fever (>100° F)
- Anorexia
- N & V
- ↑↓ Pulse & ↑ BP
- ↓ Bowel Sounds
- Dehydration

Nursing Care
- Maintain Fluid & Electrolyte Balance & ↓ G.I. Distention
  - NG Suction
  - IVs (NS, LR)
  - Potassium Supp c̄ Care
  - Peristalsis ↑ ? BS
  - I & O
  - S & S Dehydration – Hypovolemia
- Prevent Complications of Immobility
  - Position with Knees Flexed
- Decrease Pain
  - Analgesics
  - Quiet Environment

C J Miller

CROHN'S DISEASE

- Familial Tendencies
- Peaks Ages 15-40 Yrs
- ? Autoimmune Factors
- Nausea & Vomiting

- Severe Diarrhea
- Low Grade Fever
- Bloody Stools
- Weight Loss
- Severe Malabsorption

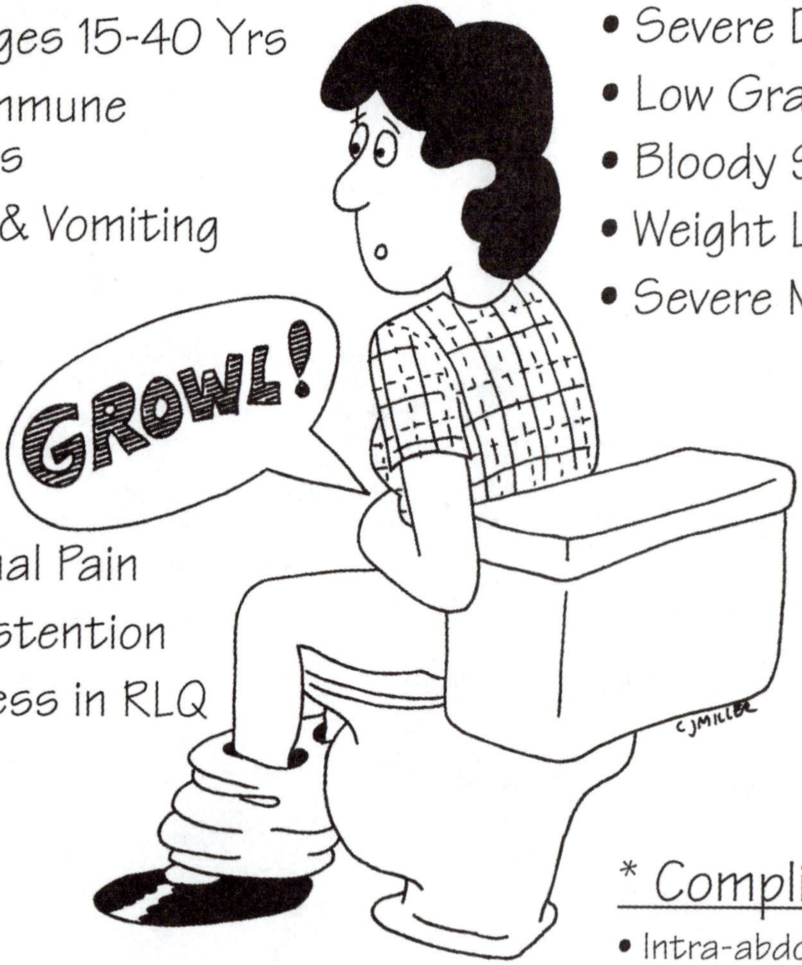

GROWL!

- Abdominal Pain and Distention
- Tenderness in RLQ

* Complications *
- Intra-abdominal Abscesses
- Intestinal Fistulas
- Peritonitis
- Development of Fistulas

* Later S & S's *
- Dehydration
- Electrolyte Imbalance
- Anemia

CJMILLER

HEPATIC ENCEPHALOPATHY

HEPATIC COMA

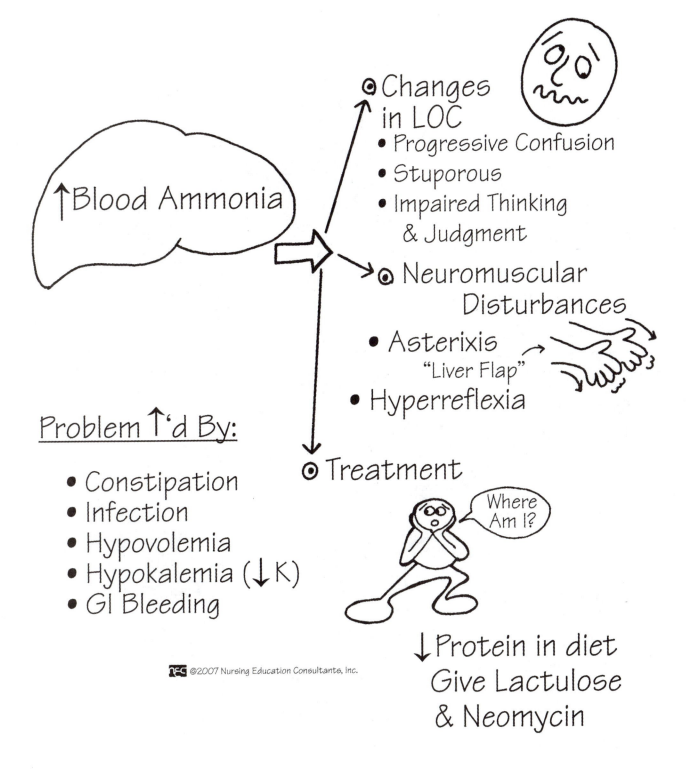

⊙ Changes in LOC
- Progressive Confusion
- Stuporous
- Impaired Thinking & Judgment

↑Blood Ammonia

⊙ Neuromuscular Disturbances
- Asterixis "Liver Flap"
- Hyperreflexia

Problem ↑'d By:
- Constipation
- Infection
- Hypovolemia
- Hypokalemia (↓K)
- GI Bleeding

⊙ Treatment

Where Am I?

↓Protein in diet
Give Lactulose
& Neomycin

CIRRHOSIS:
LATER CLINICAL MANIFESTATIONS

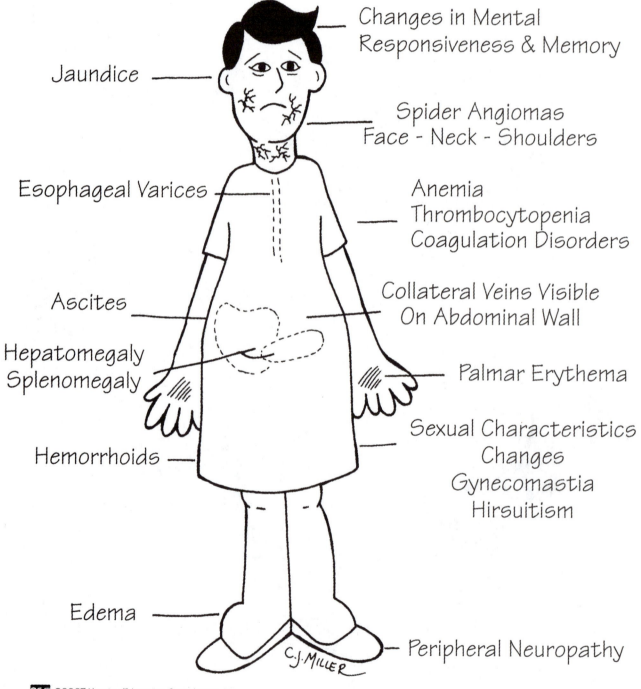

Changes in Mental Responsiveness & Memory

Jaundice

Spider Angiomas Face - Neck - Shoulders

Esophageal Varices

Anemia Thrombocytopenia Coagulation Disorders

Ascites

Collateral Veins Visible On Abdominal Wall

Hepatomegaly Splenomegaly

Palmar Erythema

Hemorrhoids

Sexual Characteristics Changes Gynecomastia Hirsuitism

Edema

Peripheral Neuropathy

C.J. MILLER

CHOLECYSTITIS

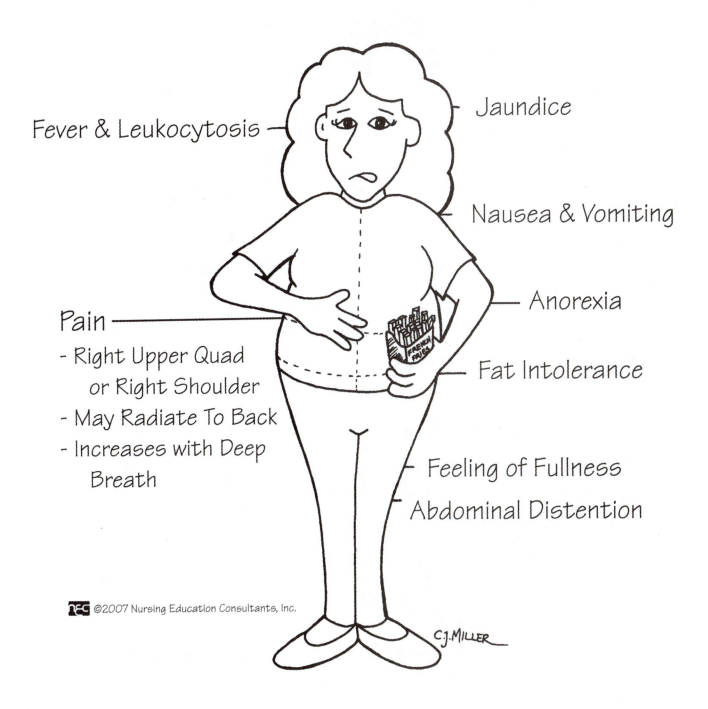

Fever & Leukocytosis

Jaundice

Nausea & Vomiting

Anorexia

Pain
- Right Upper Quad
  or Right Shoulder
- May Radiate To Back
- Increases with Deep
  Breath

Fat Intolerance

Feeling of Fullness

Abdominal Distention

C.J.MILLER

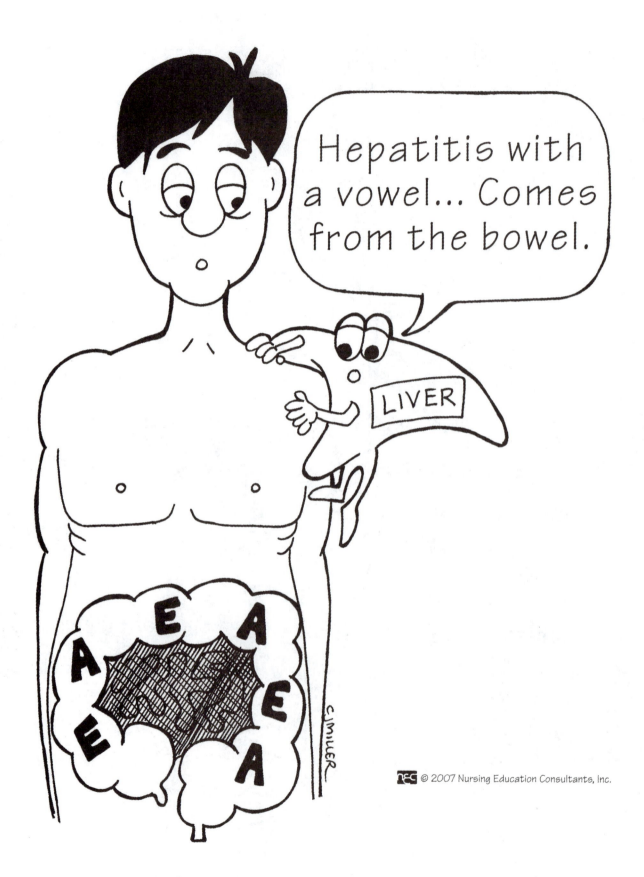

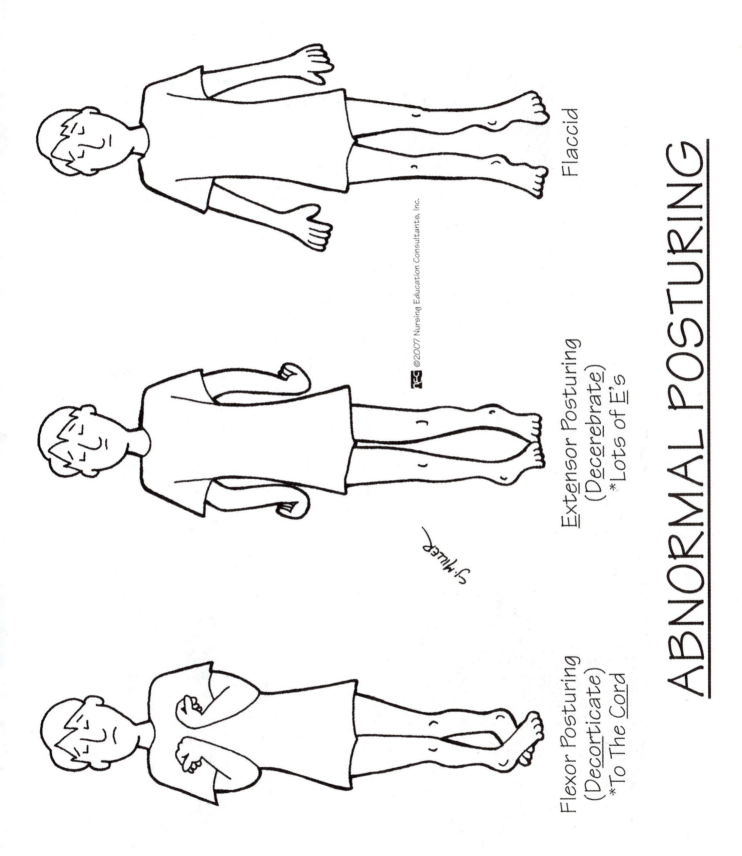

ABNORMAL POSTURING

Flaccid

Extensor Posturing
(De<u>cere</u>brate)
*Lots of <u>E</u>'s

Flexor Posturing
(De<u>cort</u>icate)
*To The <u>Cord</u>

S.J. MILLER

©2007 Nursing Education Consultants, Inc.

CRANIAL NERVE MNEMONIC

S = Sensory	M = Motor	B = Both

O	Olfactory	O	On	S	Some
O	Optic	O	Old	S	Say
O	Oculomotor	O	Olympus	M	Marry
T	Trochlear	T	Towering	M	Money
T	Trigeminal	T	Tops	B	But
A	Abducens	A	A	M	My
F	Facial	F	Finn	B	Brother
A	Acoustic	A	And	S	Says
G	Glossopharyngeal	G	German	B	Bad
V	Vagus Nerve	V	Viewed	B	Business
S	Spinal	S	Some	M	Marry
H	Hypoglossal	H	Hops	M	Money

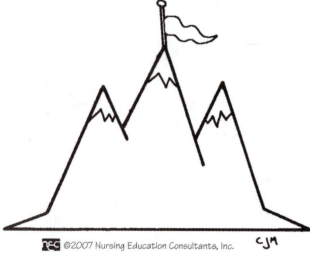

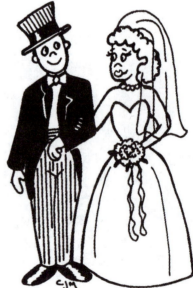

INCREASED INTRACRANIAL PRESSURE

- Changes in LOC

- Eyes
  - Papilledema
  - Pupillary Changes
  - Impaired
    Eye Movement

- Posturing
  - Decerebrate
  - Decorticate
  - Flaccid

- Decreased
  Motor Function
  - Change in Motor Ability
  - Posturing

- Headache

- Seizures
  - Impaired Sensory
    & Motor Function

- Changes in
  Vital Signs:
  - Cushing's Triad:
    - ↑ Systolic B/P
    - ↓ Pulse
    - Altered
      Resp Pattern

- Vomiting

- Changes in Speech

©2007 Nursing Education Consultants, Inc.

◎ Infants:
- Bulging Fontanels
- Cranial Suture Separation
- ↑ Head Circumference
- High Pitched Cry

INCREASED INTRACRANIAL PRESSURE
(IICP)

(Symptoms Of IICP Are Opposite Of Shock)

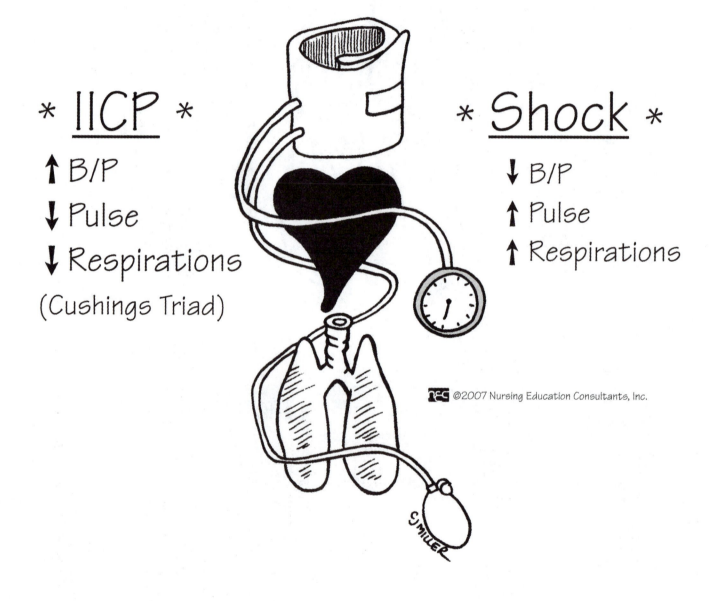

* IICP *

↑ B/P
↓ Pulse
↓ Respirations

(Cushings Triad)

* Shock *

↓ B/P
↑ Pulse
↑ Respirations

@2007 Nursing Education Consultants, Inc.

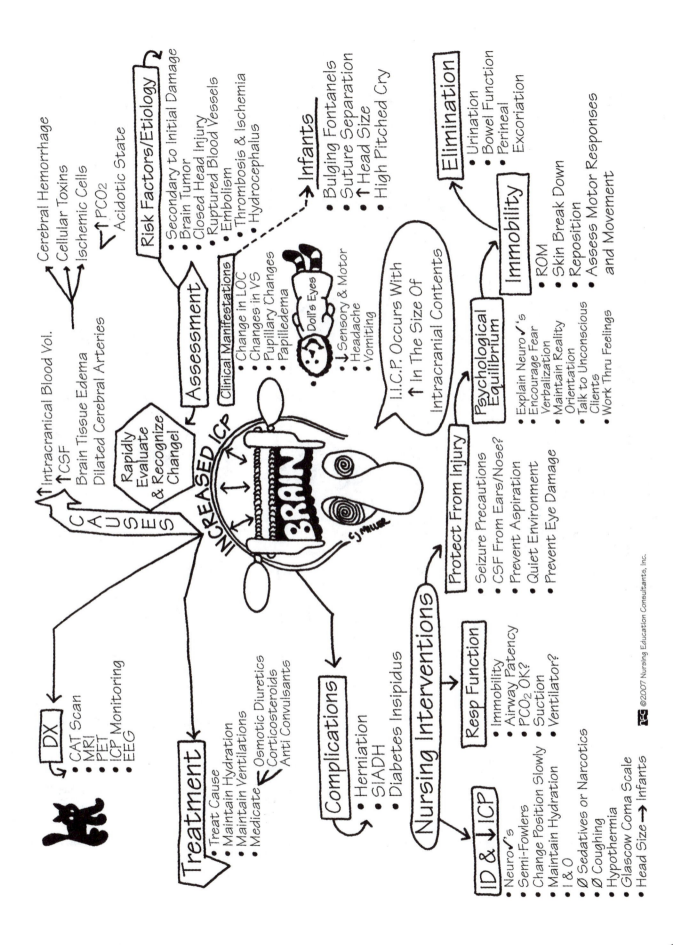

INCREASED ICP

BRAIN

S.J. Miller

↑Intracranical Blood Vol.
↑CSF
Brain Tissue Edema
Dilated Cerebral Arteries

Cerebral Hemorrhage
Cellular Toxins
Ischemic Cells
↑PCO₂
↓Acidotic State

Risk Factors/Etiology
• Secondary to Initial Damage
• Brain Tumor
• Closed Head Injury
• Ruptured Blood Vessels
• Embolism
• Thrombosis & Ischemia
• Hydrocephalus

Infants
• Bulging Fontanels
• Suture Separation
• ↑Head Size
• High Pitched Cry

Elimination
• Urination
• Bowel Function
• Perineal Excoriation

Immobility
• ROM
• Skin Break Down
• Reposition
• Assess Motor Responses and Movement

Assessment

Clinical Manifestations
• Change in LOC
• Changes in VS
• Pupillary Changes
• Papilledema

Doll's Eyes
→ Sensory & Motor
• Headache
• Vomiting

I.I.C.P. Occurs With ↑ In The Size Of Intracranial Contents

Psychological Equilibrium
• Explain Neuro ✓'s
• Encourage Fear Verbalization
• Maintain Reality Orientation
• Talk to Unconscious Clients
• Work Thru Feelings

Rapidly Evaluate & Recognize Change!

CAUSES

DX
• CAT Scan
• MRI
• PET
• ICP Monitoring
• EEG

Treatment
• Treat Cause
• Maintain Hydration
• Maintain Ventilations
• Medicate — Osmotic Diuretics
   Corticosteroids
   Anti Convulsants

Complications
• Herniation
• SIADH
• Diabetes Insipidus

Nursing Interventions

Resp Function
• Immobility
• Airway Patency
• PCO₂ OK?
• Suction
• Ventilator?

Protect From Injury
• Seizure Precautions
• CSF From Ears/Nose?
• Prevent Aspiration
• Quiet Environment
• Prevent Eye Damage

ID & ↓ICP
• Neuro ✓'s
• Semi-Fowlers
• Change Position Slowly
• Maintain Hydration
• I & O
• Ø Sedatives or Narcotics
• Ø Coughing
• Hypothermia
• Glascow Coma Scale
• Head Size → Infants

©2007 Nursing Education Consultants, Inc.

Stroke
BRAIN ACCIDENT - CVA

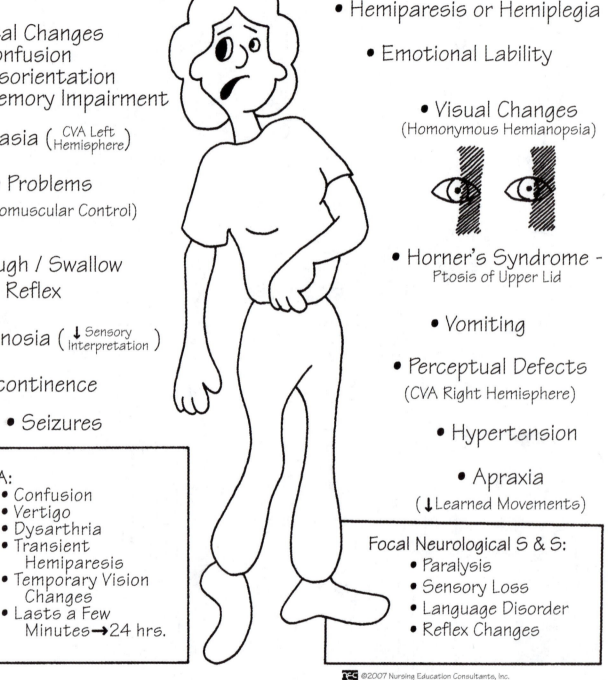

- Headache

- Mental Changes
  - Confusion
  - Disorientation
  - Memory Impairment

- Aphasia (CVA Left Hemisphere)

- Resp Problems
  (↓ Neuromuscular Control)

- ↓ Cough / Swallow Reflex

- Agnosia (↓ Sensory Interpretation)

- Incontinence

- Seizures

- Hemiparesis or Hemiplegia

- Emotional Lability

- Visual Changes
  (Homonymous Hemianopsia)

- Horner's Syndrome -
  Ptosis of Upper Lid

- Vomiting

- Perceptual Defects
  (CVA Right Hemisphere)

- Hypertension

- Apraxia
  (↓ Learned Movements)

TIA:
- Confusion
- Vertigo
- Dysarthria
- Transient Hemiparesis
- Temporary Vision Changes
- Lasts a Few Minutes → 24 hrs.

Focal Neurological S & S:
- Paralysis
- Sensory Loss
- Language Disorder
- Reflex Changes

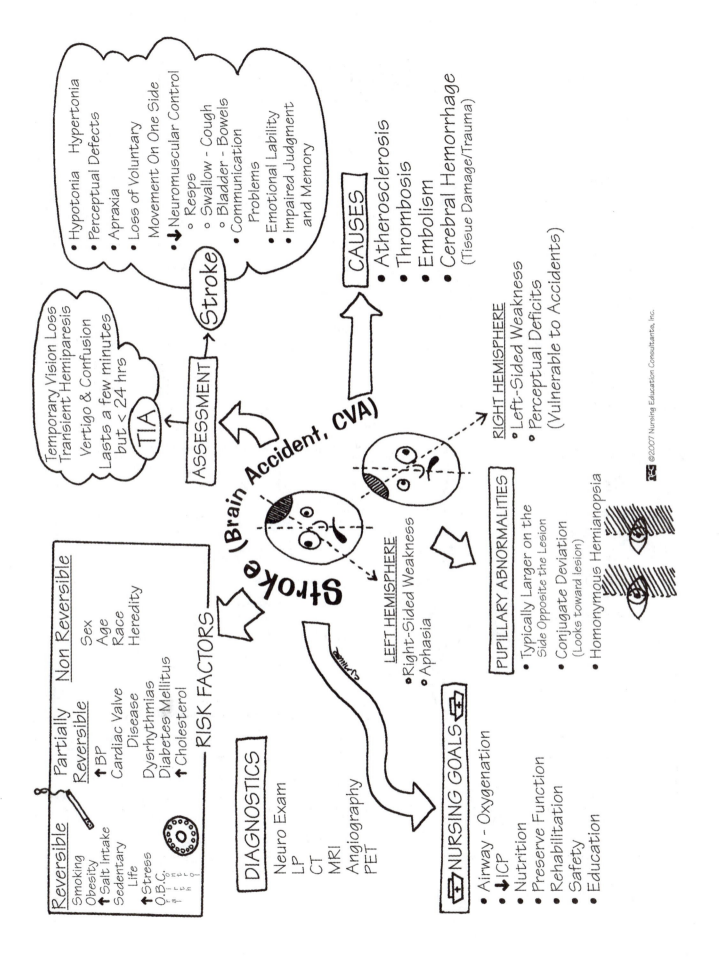

Stroke (Brain Accident, CVA)

Stroke
- Hypotonia Hypertonia
- Perceptual Defects
- Apraxia
- Loss of Voluntary Movement On One Side
- ➡ Neuromuscular Control
  - Resps
  - Swallow - Cough
  - Bladder - Bowels
  - Communication Problems
- Emotional Lability
- Impaired Judgment and Memory

ASSESSMENT

TIA
- Temporary Vision Loss
- Transient Hemiparesis
- Vertigo & Confusion
- Lasts a few minutes but < 24 hrs

CAUSES
- Atherosclerosis
- Thrombosis
- Embolism
- Cerebral Hemorrhage (Tissue Damage/Trauma)

RIGHT HEMISPHERE
- Left-Sided Weakness
- Perceptual Deficits (Vulnerable to Accidents)

LEFT HEMISPHERE
- Right-Sided Weakness
- Aphasia

PUPILLARY ABNORMALITIES
- Typically Larger on the Side Opposite the Lesion
- Conjugate Deviation (Looks toward lesion)
- Homonymous Hemianopsia

RISK FACTORS

Reversible
- Smoking
- Obesity
- ⬆ Salt Intake
- Sedentary Life
- ⬆ Stress
- O.B.C. (Oral Birth Control)

Partially Reversible
- ⬆ BP
- Cardiac Valve Disease
- Dysrhythmias
- Diabetes Mellitus
- ⬆ Cholesterol

Non Reversible
- Sex
- Age
- Race
- Heredity

DIAGNOSTICS
- Neuro Exam
- LP
- CT
- MRI
- Angiography
- PET

NURSING GOALS
- Airway - Oxygenation
- ➡ ICP
- Nutrition
- Preserve Function
- Rehabilitation
- Safety
- Education

©2007 Nursing Education Consultants, Inc.

FAST Recognition Of A Stroke

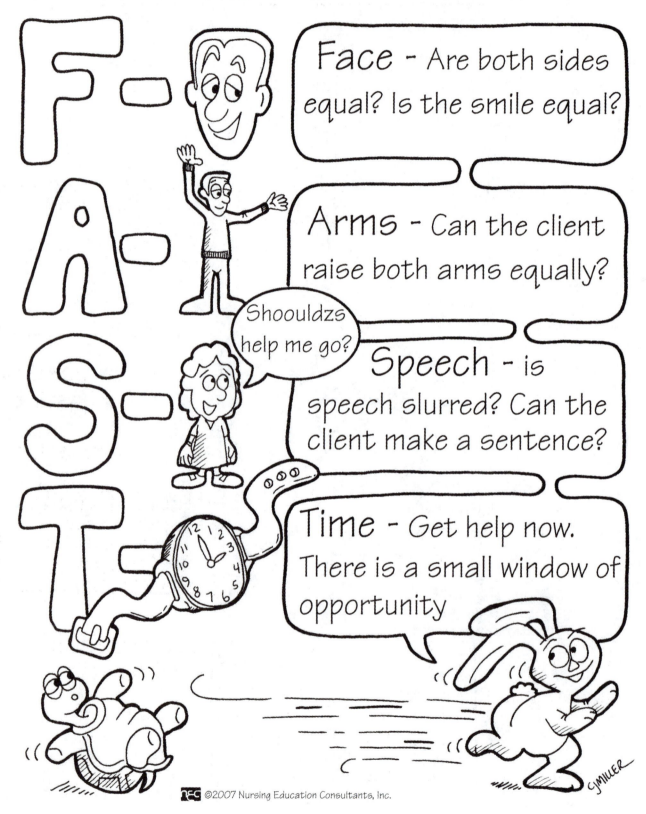

F- Face - Are both sides equal? Is the smile equal?

A- Arms - Can the client raise both arms equally?

Shoouldzs help me go?

S- Speech - is speech slurred? Can the client make a sentence?

T- Time - Get help now. There is a small window of opportunity

PARKINSON'S DISEASE

- Onset usually gradual, after age 50. (Slowly progressive)

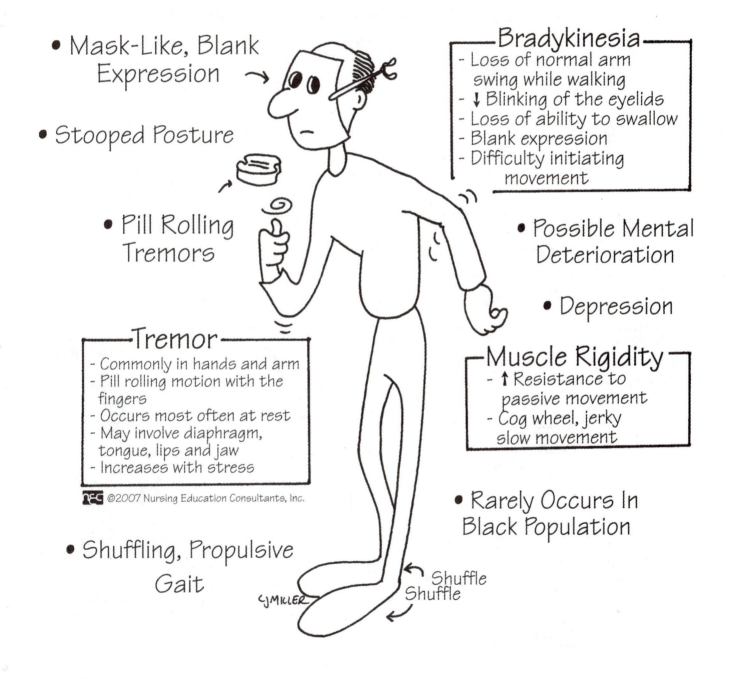

- Mask-Like, Blank Expression

- Stooped Posture

- Pill Rolling Tremors

Bradykinesia
- Loss of normal arm swing while walking
- ↓ Blinking of the eyelids
- Loss of ability to swallow
- Blank expression
- Difficulty initiating movement

- Possible Mental Deterioration

- Depression

Tremor
- Commonly in hands and arm
- Pill rolling motion with the fingers
- Occurs most often at rest
- May involve diaphragm, tongue, lips and jaw
- Increases with stress

Muscle Rigidity
- ↑ Resistance to passive movement
- Cog wheel, jerky slow movement

- Rarely Occurs In Black Population

- Shuffling, Propulsive Gait

Shuffle Shuffle

CJMILLER

Bell's Palsy

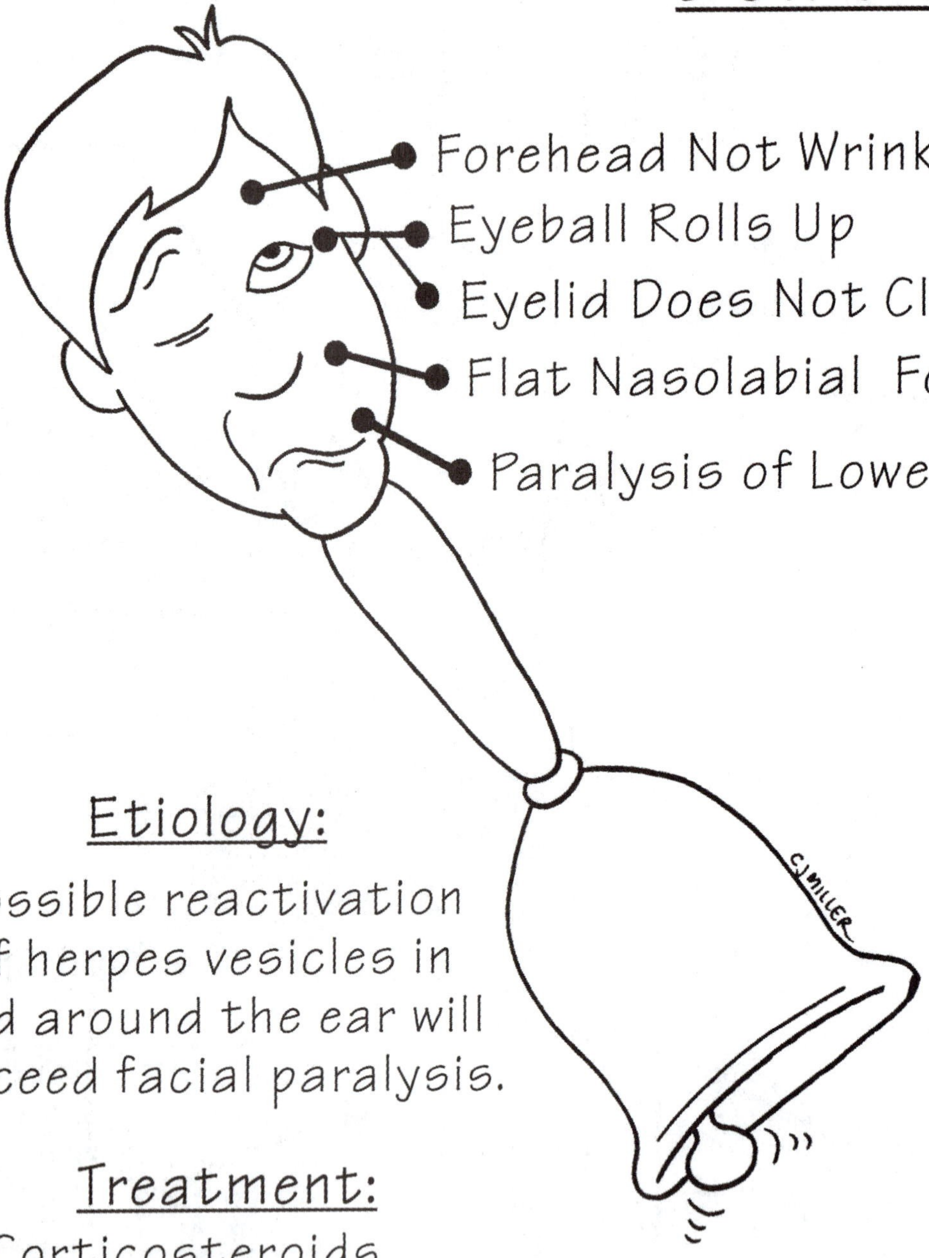

Forehead Not Wrinkled

Eyeball Rolls Up

Eyelid Does Not Close

Flat Nasolabial Fold

Paralysis of Lower Face

Etiology:

Possible reactivation of herpes vesicles in and around the ear will proceed facial paralysis.

Treatment:

- Corticosteroids
- Antivirals
- Time - 85% Full Recovery In 6 Months

Facial Nerve Involvement

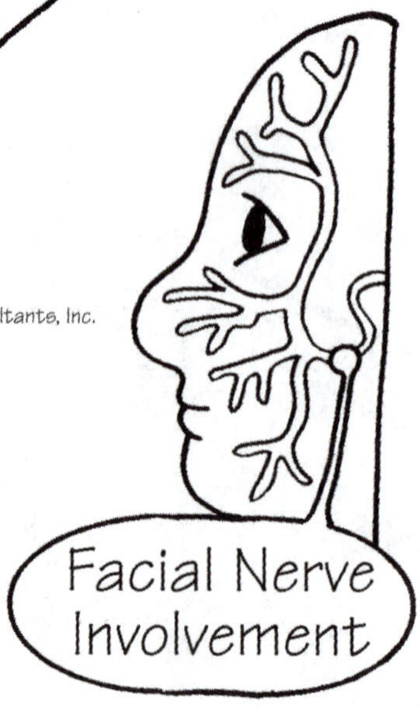

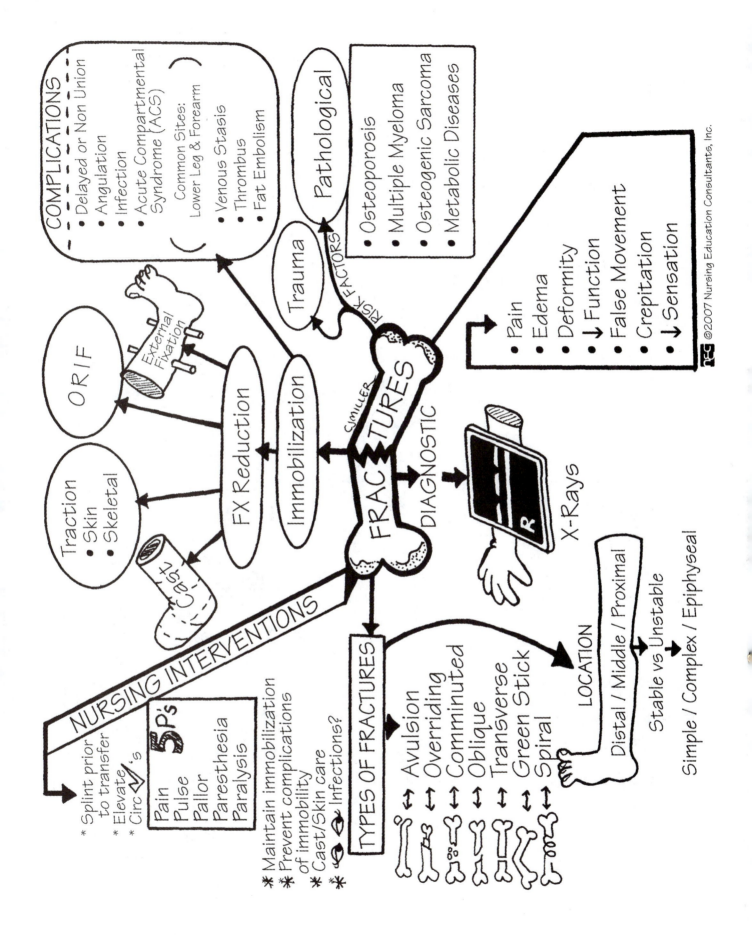

FRACTURES

COMPLICATIONS
- Delayed or Non Union
- Angulation
- Infection
- Acute Compartmental Syndrome (ACS)
  Common Sites: Lower Leg & Forearm
- Venous Stasis
- Thrombus
- Fat Embolism

Pathological
- Osteoporosis
- Multiple Myeloma
- Osteogenic Sarcoma
- Metabolic Diseases

Trauma

RISK FACTORS

DIAGNOSTIC
- Pain
- Edema
- Deformity
- ↑ Function
- False Movement
- Crepitation
- ↓ Sensation

X-Rays

ORIF

External Fixation

Traction
- Skin
- Skeletal

FX Reduction

Immobilization

Cast

NURSING INTERVENTIONS

* Splint prior to transfer
* Elevate
* Circ ✓'s

5 P's
Pain
Pulse
Pallor
Paresthesia
Paralysis

* Maintain immobilization
** Prevent complications of immobility
** Cast/Skin care
** Infections?

TYPES OF FRACTURES
- Avulsion
- Overriding
- Comminuted
- Oblique
- Transverse
- Green Stick
- Spiral

LOCATION
Distal / Middle / Proximal

Stable vs Unstable

Simple / Complex / Epiphyseal

©2007 Nursing Education Consultants, Inc.

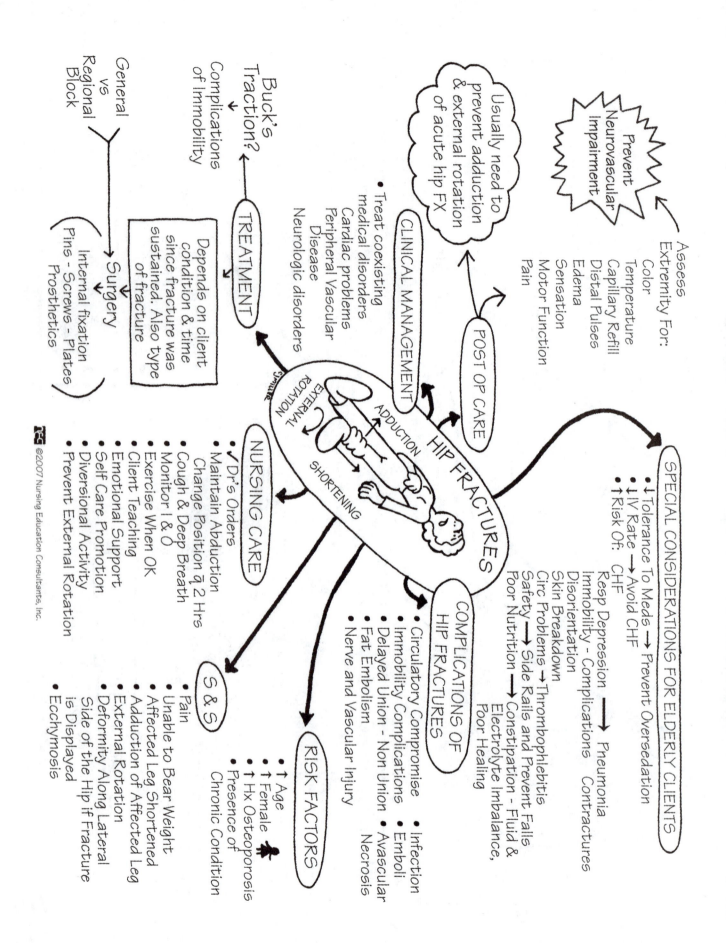

HIP FRACTURES

Prevent Neurovascular Impairment

Assess Extremity For:
- Color
- Temperature
- Capillary Refill
- Distal Pulses
- Edema
- Sensation
- Motor Function
- Pain

Usually need to prevent adduction & external rotation of acute hip FX

POST OP CARE

CLINICAL MANAGEMENT
- Treat coexisting medical disorders
  - Cardiac problems
  - Peripheral Vascular Disease
  - Neurologic disorders

TREATMENT

Complications of Immobility

Buck's Traction?

Depends on client condition & time since fracture was sustained. Also type of fracture

Surgery
- Internal fixation (Pins - Screws - Plates)
- Prosthetics

General vs Regional Block

EXTERNAL ROTATION
ADDUCTION
SHORTENING

NURSING CARE
- ✓ Dr's Orders
- Maintain Abduction
- Change Position q 2 Hrs
- Cough & Deep Breath
- Monitor I & O
- Exercise When OK
- Client Teaching
- Emotional Support
- Self Care Promotion
- Diversional Activity
- Prevent External Rotation

S & S
- Pain
- Unable to Bear Weight
- Affected Leg Shortened
- Adduction of Affected Leg
- External Rotation
- Deformity Along Lateral Side of the Hip if Fracture is Displayed
- Ecchymosis

RISK FACTORS
- ↑ Age
- ↑ Female
- ↑ Hx Osteoporosis
- Presence of Chronic Condition

COMPLICATIONS OF HIP FRACTURES
- Circulatory Compromise
- Immobility Complications
- Delayed Union - Non Union
- Fat Embolism
- Nerve and Vascular Injury
- Infection
- Emboli
- Avascular Necrosis

SPECIAL CONSIDERATIONS FOR ELDERLY CLIENTS
- ↓ Tolerance To Meds →
- ↓ IV Rate → Avoid CHF
- ↑ Risk Of: CHF
  - Resp Depression → Prevent Oversedation
  - Immobility - Complications → Pneumonia Contractures
  - Disorientation
  - Skin Breakdown
  - Circ Problems → Thrombophlebitis
  - Safety → Side Rails and Prevent Falls
  - Poor Nutrition → Constipation - Fluid & Electrolyte Imbalance, Poor Healing

NURSING CARE FOR SPRAINS AND STRAINS

R Rest
I Ice
C Compression
E Elevation

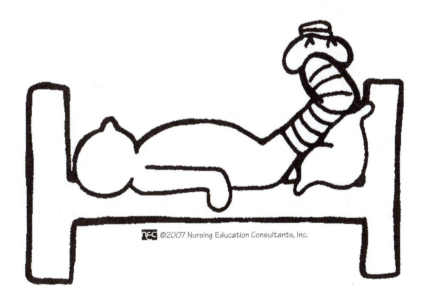

©2007 Nursing Education Consultants, Inc.

CARE OF CLIENT IN TRACTION

T Temperature < Extremity Infection

R Ropes Hang Freely

A Alignment

C Circulation Check (5 P's)

T Type & Location of Fracture

I Increase Fluid Intake

O Overhead Trapeze

N No Weights On Bed Or Floor

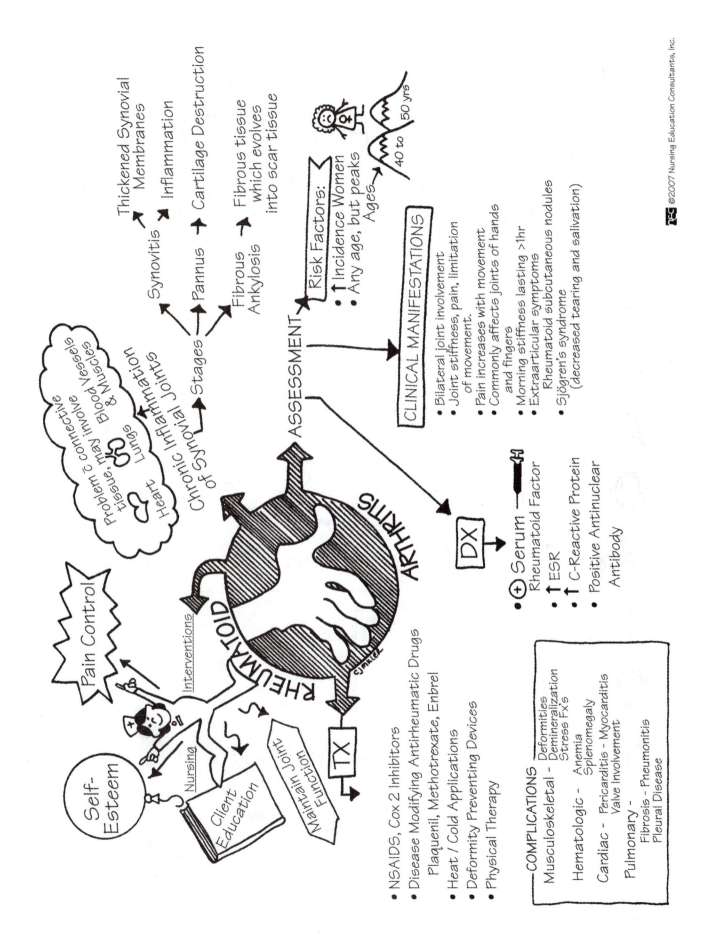

RHEUMATOID ARTHRITIS

Chronic Inflammation of Synovial Joints

Problem c̄ connective tissue, may involve Blood Vessels & Muscles, Lungs, Heart

Stages:
- Synovitis → Thickened Synovial Membranes, Inflammation
- Pannus → ↑ Cartilage Destruction
- Fibrous Ankylosis → Fibrous tissue which evolves into scar tissue

ASSESSMENT

Risk Factors:
- ↑ Incidence Women
- Any age, but peaks Ages — 40 to 50 yrs

CLINICAL MANIFESTATIONS
- Bilateral joint involvement
- Joint stiffness, pain, limitation of movement.
- Pain increases with movement.
- Commonly affects joints of hands and fingers
- Morning stiffness lasting >1hr
- Extraarticular symptoms
- Rheumatoid subcutaneous nodules
- Sjögren's syndrome (decreased tearing and salivation)

DX
- ⊕ Serum Rheumatoid Factor
- ↑ ESR
- ↑ C-Reactive Protein
- Positive Antinuclear Antibody

TX
- NSAIDS, Cox 2 Inhibitors
- Disease Modifying Antirheumatic Drugs Plaquenil, Methotrexate, Enbrel
- Heat / Cold Applications
- Deformity Preventing Devices
- Physical Therapy

Nursing
- Client Education
- Maintain Joint Function
- Self-Esteem
- Pain Control

Interventions

COMPLICATIONS
- Musculoskeletal – Deformities, Demineralization, Stress Fx's
- Hematologic – Anemia, Splenomegaly
- Cardiac – Pericarditis – Myocarditis, Valve Involvement
- Pulmonary – Fibrosis – Pneumonitis, Pleural Disease

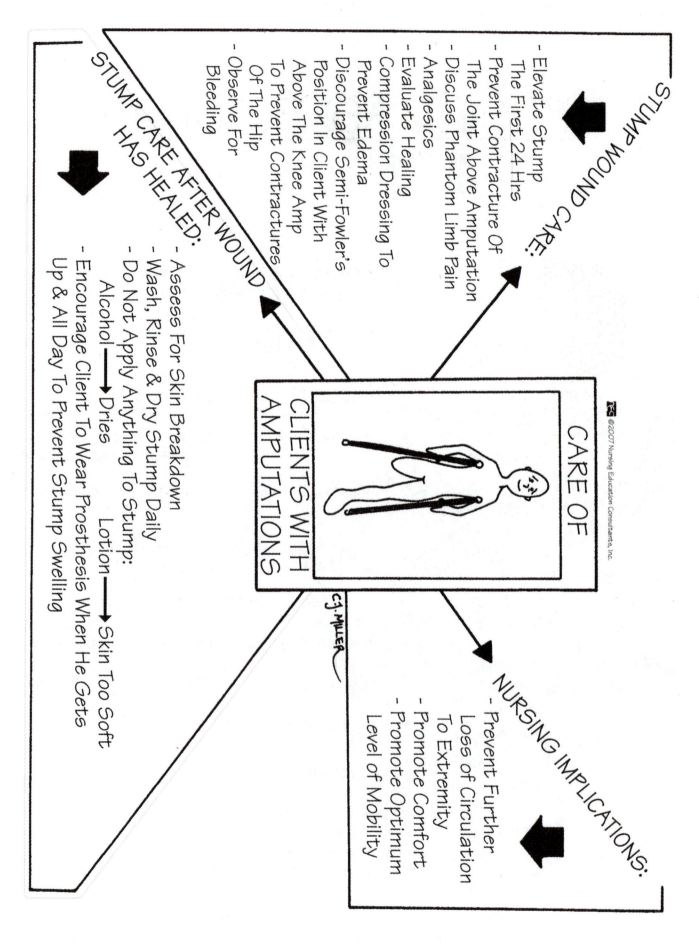

CARE OF

CLIENTS WITH AMPUTATIONS

STUMP WOUND CARE:

- Elevate Stump
  The First 24 Hrs
- Prevent Contracture Of
  The Joint Above Amputation
- Discuss Phantom Limb Pain
- Analgesics
- Evaluate Healing
- Compression Dressing To
  Prevent Edema
- Discourage Semi-Fowler's
  Position In Client With
  Above The Knee Amp
  To Prevent Contractures
  Of The Hip
- Observe For
  Bleeding

STUMP CARE AFTER WOUND HAS HEALED:

- Assess For Skin Breakdown
- Wash, Rinse & Dry Stump Daily
- Do Not Apply Anything To Stump:
  Alcohol ➝ Dries
  Lotion ➝ Skin Too Soft
- Encourage Client To Wear Prosthesis When He Gets
  Up & All Day To Prevent Stump Swelling

NURSING IMPLICATIONS:

- Prevent Further
  Loss of Circulation
  To Extremity
- Promote Comfort
- Promote Optimum
  Level of Mobility

C.J. MILLER

POST MASTECTOMY

NURSING CARE

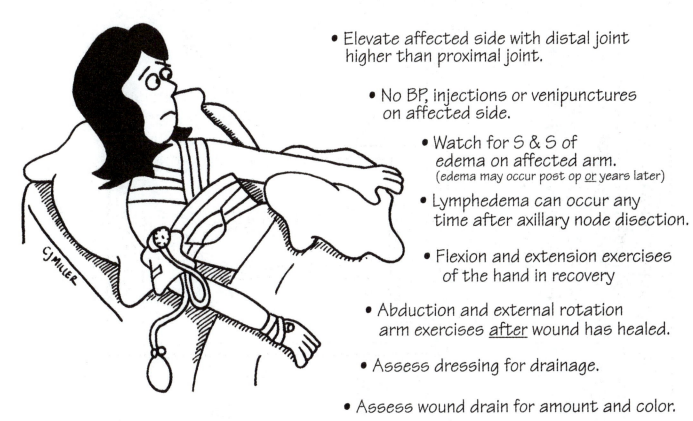

• Elevate affected side with distal joint higher than proximal joint.

• No BP, injections or venipunctures on affected side.

• Watch for S & S of edema on affected arm. (edema may occur post op <u>or</u> years later)

• Lymphedema can occur any time after axillary node disection.

• Flexion and extension exercises of the hand in recovery

• Abduction and external rotation arm exercises <u>after</u> wound has healed.

• Assess dressing for drainage.

• Assess wound drain for amount and color.

• Provide privacy when client looks at incision.

• Chemotherapy.

• Radiation therapy.

• Psychological concerns:
   Altered body image
   Altered sexuality
   Fear of disease outcome

TURP
(Transurethral Resection of the Prostate)

• Continuous or Intermittent Bladder Irrigation (C.B.I.)
Murphy Drip

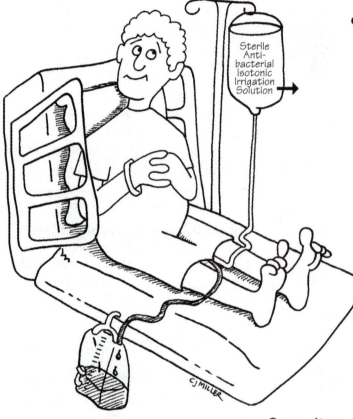

Sterile Anti-bacterial Isotonic Irrigation Solution →

• Close observation of drainage system - (↑Bladder Distention causes Pain & Bleeding).

• Maintain Catheter Patency

• Bladder Spasms

• Pain Control: Analgesics & ↓ Activity first 24 hours.

• Avoid straining with BM's ↑ Fiber diet & Laxatives.

CJ MILLER

• Complications:
  • Hemorrhage - Bleeding should gradually ↓ to light pink in 24 hrs.
  • Urinary Incontinence - Kegal Exercises
  • Infections - ↑ Fluids
  • Prevent Deep Vein Thrombosis
    • Sequential compression stockings
    • Low dose heparin
    • Discourage sitting for prolonged periods

URINARY TRACT INFECTION: (U.T.I)

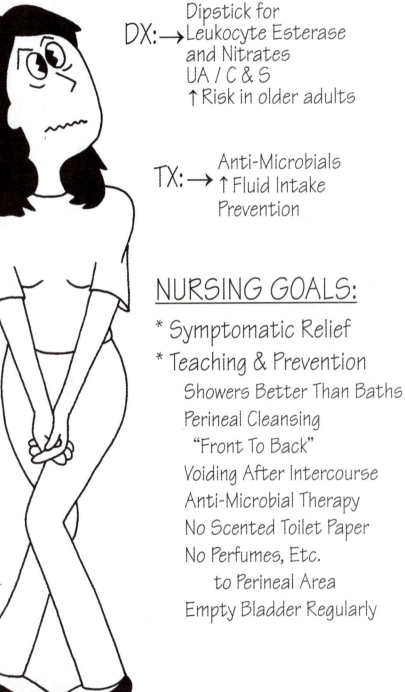

CYSTITIS:
Frequency
Urgency
Suprapubic Pain
Dysuria
Hematuria
Fever
Confusion
   in Older Adults

PYELONEPHRITIS:
Flank Pain
Dysuria
Pain At Costovertebral
   Angle
Same S & S as Cystitis

DX: → Dipstick for
Leukocyte Esterase
and Nitrates
UA / C & S
↑ Risk in older adults

TX: → Anti-Microbials
↑ Fluid Intake
Prevention

NURSING GOALS:
* Symptomatic Relief
* Teaching & Prevention
   Showers Better Than Baths
   Perineal Cleansing
    "Front To Back"
   Voiding After Intercourse
   Anti-Microbial Therapy
   No Scented Toilet Paper
   No Perfumes, Etc.
    to Perineal Area
   Empty Bladder Regularly

CJMILLER

113

RENAL CALCULI

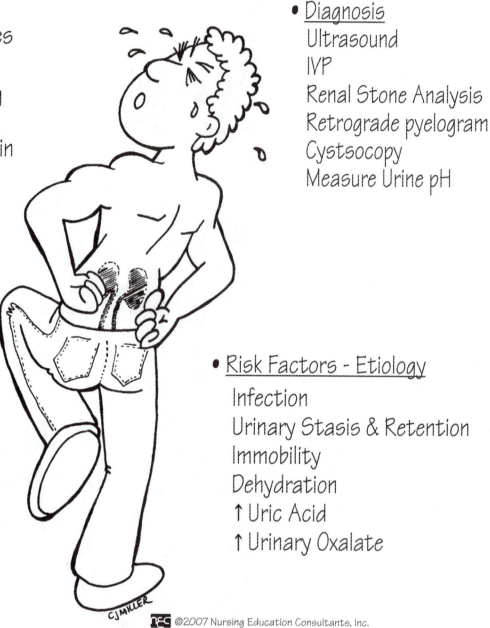

- ↑ Incidence in Males

- Nausea & Vomiting

- Agonizing Flank Pain
  May Radiate To:
  Groin
  Testicles
  Abdominal Area

- Sharp, Sudden,
  Severe Pain:
  (May be intermittent
  depending on
  stone movement)

- Hematuria

- Dysuria

- Urinary Frequency

- <u>Diagnosis</u>
  Ultrasound
  IVP
  Renal Stone Analysis
  Retrograde pyelogram
  Cystsocopy
  Measure Urine pH

- <u>Risk Factors - Etiology</u>
  Infection
  Urinary Stasis & Retention
  Immobility
  Dehydration
  ↑ Uric Acid
  ↑ Urinary Oxalate

CJMILLER

@2007 Nursing Education Consultants, Inc.

CHRONIC RENAL FAILURE (CRF)
- DIMINISHED RENAL RESERVE -

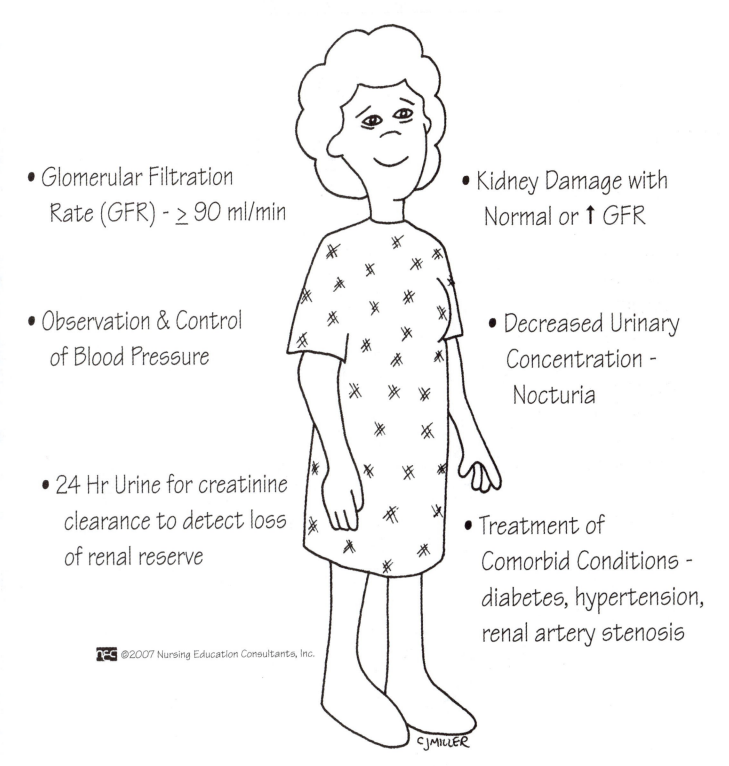

- Glomerular Filtration Rate (GFR) - ≥ 90 ml/min

- Observation & Control of Blood Pressure

- 24 Hr Urine for creatinine clearance to detect loss of renal reserve

- Kidney Damage with Normal or ↑ GFR

- Decreased Urinary Concentration - Nocturia

- Treatment of Comorbid Conditions - diabetes, hypertension, renal artery stenosis

©2007 Nursing Education Consultants, Inc.

CJMILLER

CHRONIC RENAL FAILURE (CRF)
- RENAL INSUFFICIENCY -

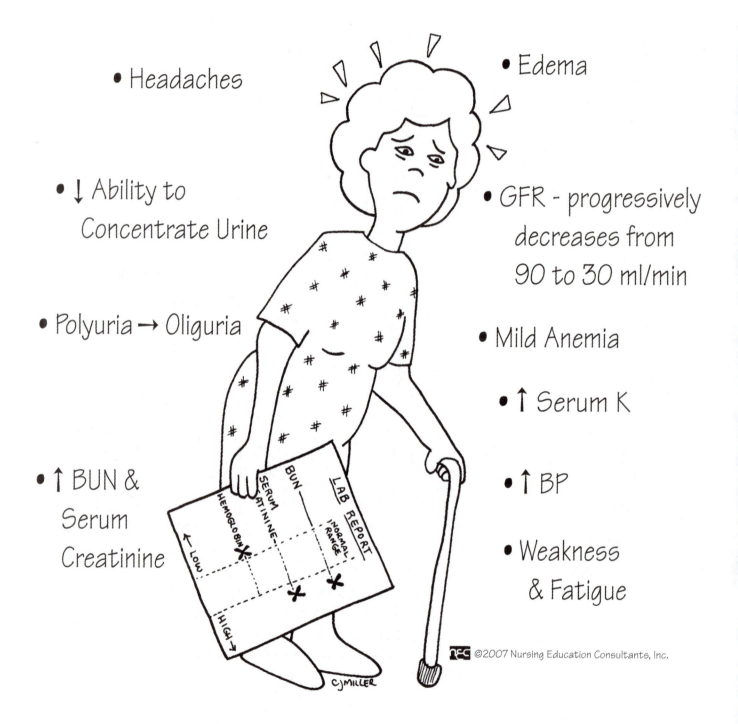

- Headaches
- ↓ Ability to Concentrate Urine
- Polyuria → Oliguria
- ↑ BUN & Serum Creatinine
- Edema
- GFR - progressively decreases from 90 to 30 ml/min
- Mild Anemia
- ↑ Serum K
- ↑ BP
- Weakness & Fatigue

©2007 Nursing Education Consultants, Inc.

CJMILLER

CHRONIC RENAL FAILURE (CRF)

ESRD - END STAGE RENAL DISEASE
$\downarrow$ 15 ml/min GFR

- Neurological
  Weakness / Fatigue
  Confusion

- Cardiovascular
  $\uparrow$ BP
  Pitting Edema
  Periorbital Edema
  $\uparrow$ CVP
  Pericarditis

- Pulmonary
  SOB
  Depressed Cough
  Thick Sputum

- GI
  Ammonia Odor to Breath
  Metallic Taste
  Mouth / Gum Ulcerations
  Anorexia
  Nausea / Vomiting

- Psychological
  Withdrawn
  Behavior Changes
  Depression

- Hematological
  Anemia
  Bleeding Tendencies
  $\uparrow$ Serum K

- Musculoskeletal
  Cramps
  Renal Osteodystrophy
  Bone Pain

- Skin
  Dry Flaky
  Pruritus
  Ecchymosis
  Purpura
  Yellow-gray
  skin color

CJMILLER

┌─ Hemodialysis ─┐
Evaluate access site for:
Patency & signs of infection
DO NOT take BP or obtain
blood samples from extremity
that has access site.

PHYSIOLOGICAL CHANGES IN PREGNANCY

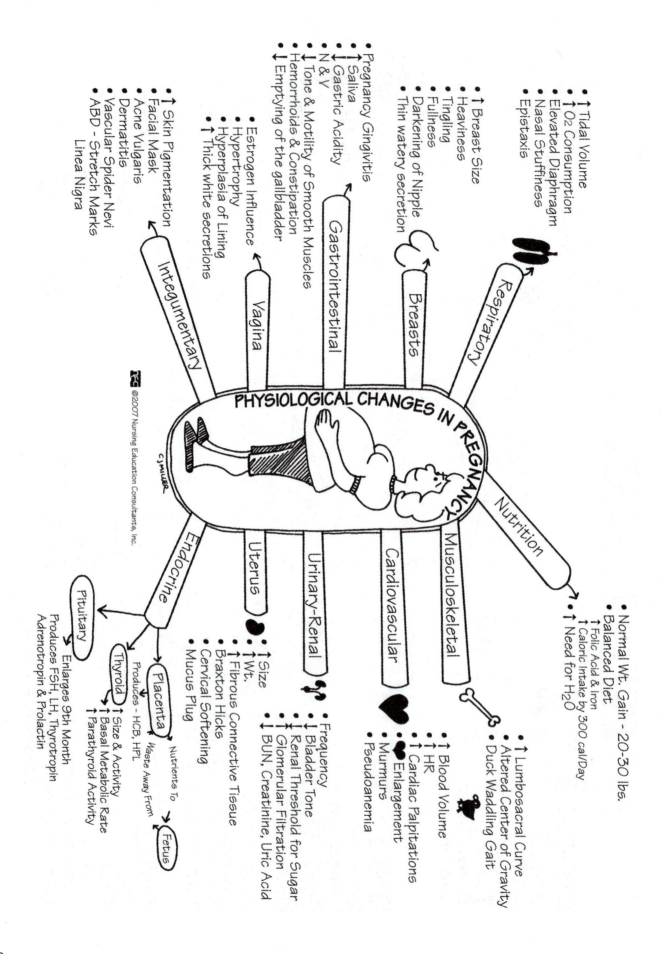

Respiratory
- ↑ Tidal Volume
- ↑ O₂ Consumption
- Elevated Diaphragm
- Nasal Stuffiness
- Epistaxis

Breasts
- ↑ Breast Size
- Heaviness
- Tingling
- Fullness
- Darkening of Nipple
- Thin watery secretion

Gastrointestinal
- Pregnancy Gingivitis
- ↑ Saliva
- ↑ Gastric Acidity
- N & V
- ↑ Tone & Motility of Smooth Muscles
- Hemorrhoids & Constipation
- ↓ Emptying of the gallbladder

Vagina
- Estrogen Influence
- Hypertrophy
- Hyperplasia of Lining
- ↑ Thick white secretions

Integumentary
- ↑ Skin Pigmentation
- Facial Mask
- Acne Vulgaris
- Dermatitis
- Vascular Spider Nevi
- ABD - Stretch Marks
- Linea Nigra

Nutrition
- Normal Wt. Gain - 20-30 lbs.
- Balanced Diet
- ↑ Folic Acid & Iron
- ↑ Caloric Intake by 300 cal/Day
- ↑ Need for H₂O

Musculoskeletal
- ↑ Lumbosacral Curve
- Altered Center of Gravity
- Duck Waddling Gait

Cardiovascular
- ↑ Blood Volume
- ↑ HR
- ↑ Cardiac Palpitations
- Enlargement
- Murmurs
- Pseudoanemia

Urinary-Renal
- ↑ Size
- ↑ Wt.
- ↑ Frequency
- ↓ Bladder Tone
- ↑ Renal Threshold for Sugar
- ↑ Glomerular Filtration
- ↓ BUN, Creatinine, Uric Acid

Uterus
- Braxton Hicks
- Fibrous Connective Tissue
- Cervical Softening
- Mucus Plug

Endocrine
- Placenta — Produces - HCB, HPL
  - Nutrients To / Waste Away From → Fetus
- Thyroid
  - ↑ Size & Activity
  - ↑ Basal Metabolic Rate
  - ↑ Parathyroid Activity
- Pituitary
  - Enlarges 9th Month
  - Produces FSH, LH, Thyrotropin
  - Adrenotropin & Prolactin

C.J. MILLER

PRENATAL CARE

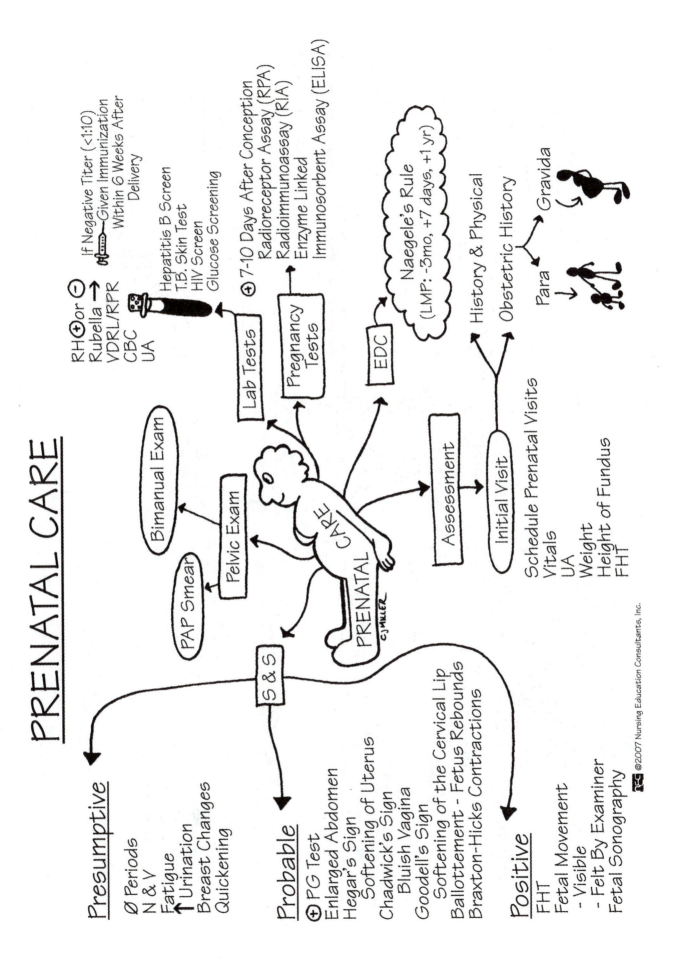

Lab Tests
- RH ⊕ or ⊖
- Rubella
- VDRL/RPR
- CBC
- UA
- Hepatitis B Screen
- T.B. Skin Test
- HIV Screen
- Glucose Screening

If Negative Titer (<1:10) — Given Immunization Within 6 Weeks After Delivery

Pregnancy Tests
- ⊕ 7-10 Days After Conception
- Radioreceptor Assay (RPA)
- Radioimmunoassay (RIA)
- Enzyme Linked Immunosorbent Assay (ELISA)

EDC

Naegele's Rule
(LMP: -3mo, +7 days, +1 yr)

- History & Physical
- Obstetric History

Gravida

Para

Assessment

Initial Visit
- Schedule Prenatal Visits
- Vitals
- UA
- Weight
- Height Of Fundus
- FHT

Bimanual Exam

Pelvic Exam

PAP Smear

PRENATAL CARE
CJMILLER

S & S

Presumptive
- Ø Periods
- N & V
- Fatigue
- ↑ Urination
- Breast Changes
- Quickening

Probable
- ⊕ PG Test
- Enlarged Abdomen
- Hegar's Sign — Softening of Uterus
- Chadwick's Sign — Bluish Vagina
- Goodell's Sign — Softening of the Cervical Lip
- Ballottement - Fetus Rebounds
- Braxton-Hicks Contractions

Positive
- FHT
- Fetal Movement
  - Visible
  - Felt By Examiner
- Fetal Sonography

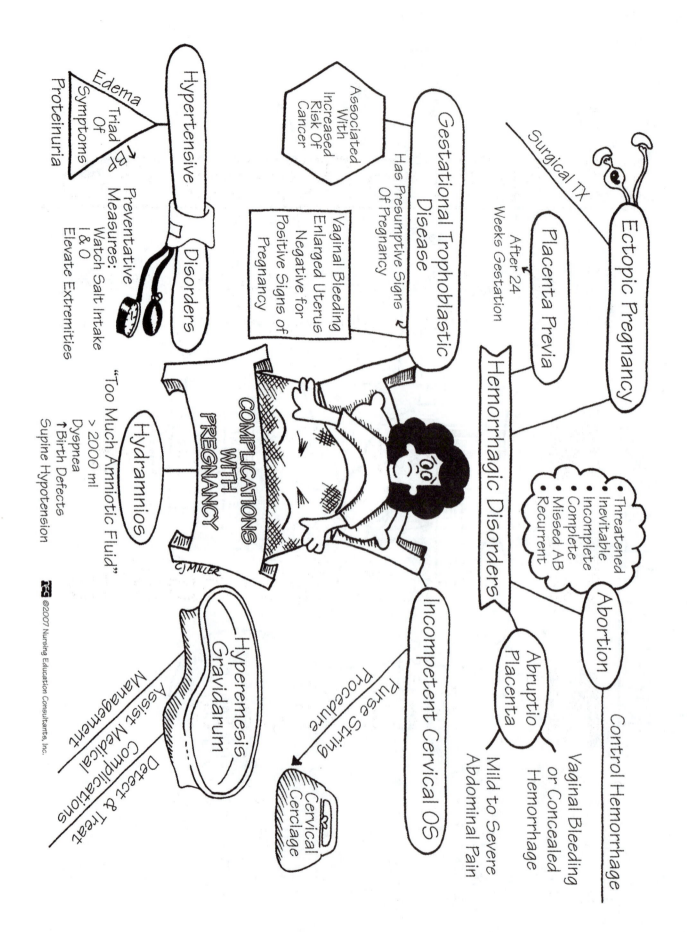

Complications with Pregnancy

Hypertensive Disorders
Triad Of Symptoms:
Edema
↑BP
Proteinuria

Preventative Measures:
Watch Salt Intake
I & O
Elevate Extremities

Gestational Trophoblastic Disease
Associated With Increased Risk Of Cancer
Has Presumptive Signs Of Pregnancy
Vaginal Bleeding
Enlarged Uterus
Negative for Positive Signs of Pregnancy

Ectopic Pregnancy
Surgical TX

Placenta Previa
After 24 Weeks Gestation

Hemorrhagic Disorders

Abortion
• Threatened
• Inevitable
• Incomplete
• Complete
• Missed AB
• Recurrent

Control Hemorrhage

Abruptio Placenta
Vaginal Bleeding or Concealed Hemorrhage
Mild to Severe Abdominal Pain

Incompetent Cervical OS
Purse String Procedure
Cervical Cerclage

Hydramnios
"Too Much Amniotic Fluid"
> 2000 ml
Dyspnea
↑Birth Defects
Supine Hypotension

Hyperemesis Gravidarum
Management
Assist Medical
Detect & Treat Complications

CJ MILLER

O.B. NON-STRESS TEST

3 Negatives in a row to interpret results
of non-stress test

N   Non-Reactive

N   Non-Stress is

N   Not Good

ASSESSMENT TESTS FOR FETAL WELL-BEING

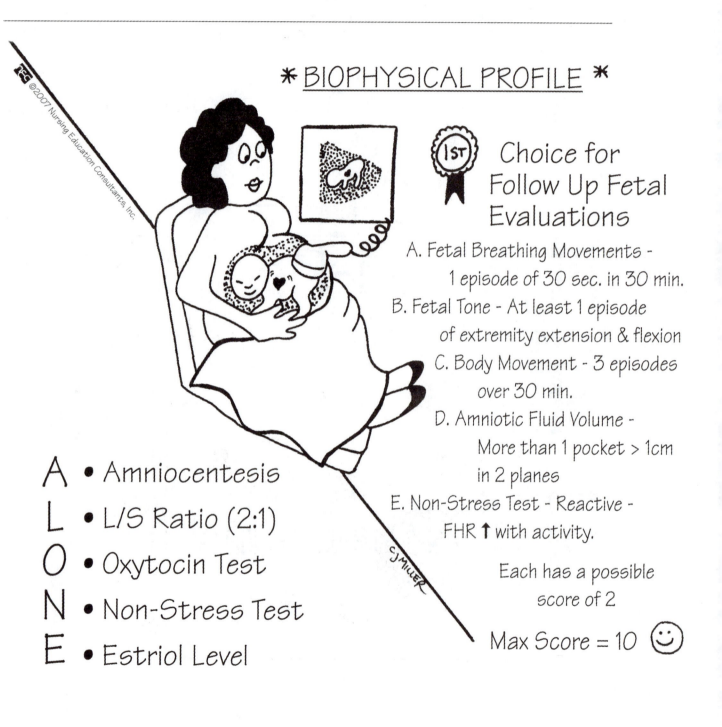

* BIOPHYSICAL PROFILE *

1st Choice for Follow Up Fetal Evaluations

A. Fetal Breathing Movements - 1 episode of 30 sec. in 30 min.

B. Fetal Tone - At least 1 episode of extremity extension & flexion

C. Body Movement - 3 episodes over 30 min.

D. Amniotic Fluid Volume - More than 1 pocket > 1cm in 2 planes

E. Non-Stress Test - Reactive - FHR ↑ with activity.

Each has a possible score of 2

Max Score = 10 ☺

A • Amniocentesis
L • L/S Ratio (2:1)
O • Oxytocin Test
N • Non-Stress Test
E • Estriol Level

HELLP Syndrome

(Preeclampsia with Liver Involvement)

Hemolysis
Elevated **L**iver Function Tests
Low **P**latelet Count

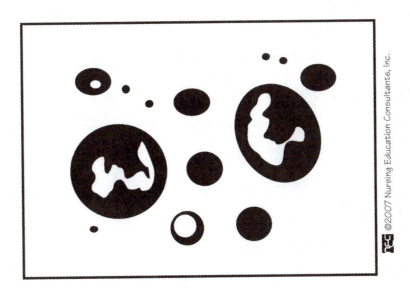

©2007 Nursing Education Consultants, Inc.

STAGES OF LABOR

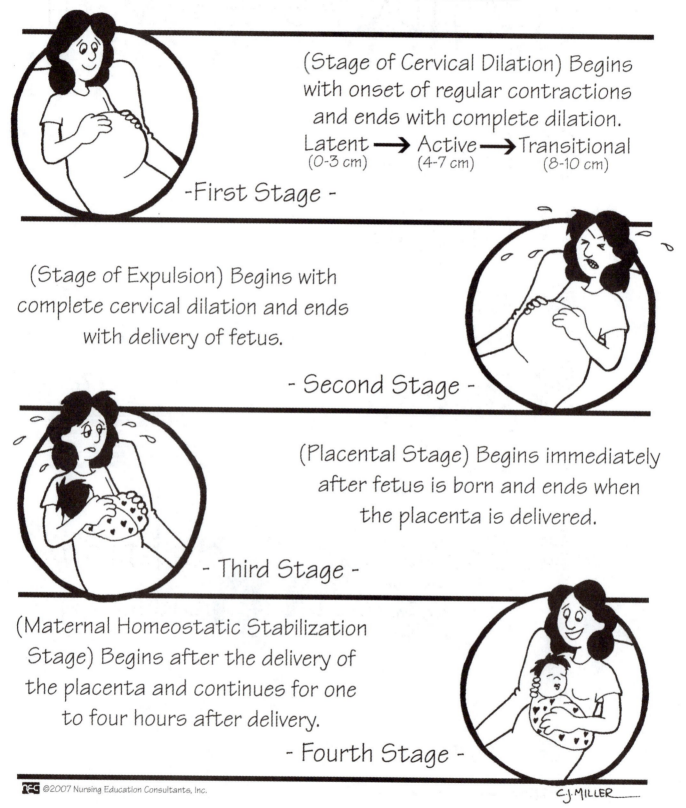

(Stage of Cervical Dilation) Begins with onset of regular contractions and ends with complete dilation.

Latent → Active → Transitional
(0-3 cm)   (4-7 cm)   (8-10 cm)

-First Stage -

(Stage of Expulsion) Begins with complete cervical dilation and ends with delivery of fetus.

- Second Stage -

(Placental Stage) Begins immediately after fetus is born and ends when the placenta is delivered.

- Third Stage -

(Maternal Homeostatic Stabilization Stage) Begins after the delivery of the placenta and continues for one to four hours after delivery.

- Fourth Stage -

C.J. MILLER

POSTPARTUM ASSESSMENT

B **B**reasts

U **U**terus

B **B**owels

B **B**ladder

L **L**ochia

E **E**pisiotomy/Laceration/
C-Section Incision

EVALUATION OF EPISIOSTOMY HEALING

R **R**edness

E **E**dema

E **E**cchymosis

D **D**ischarge, **D**rainage

A **A**pproximation

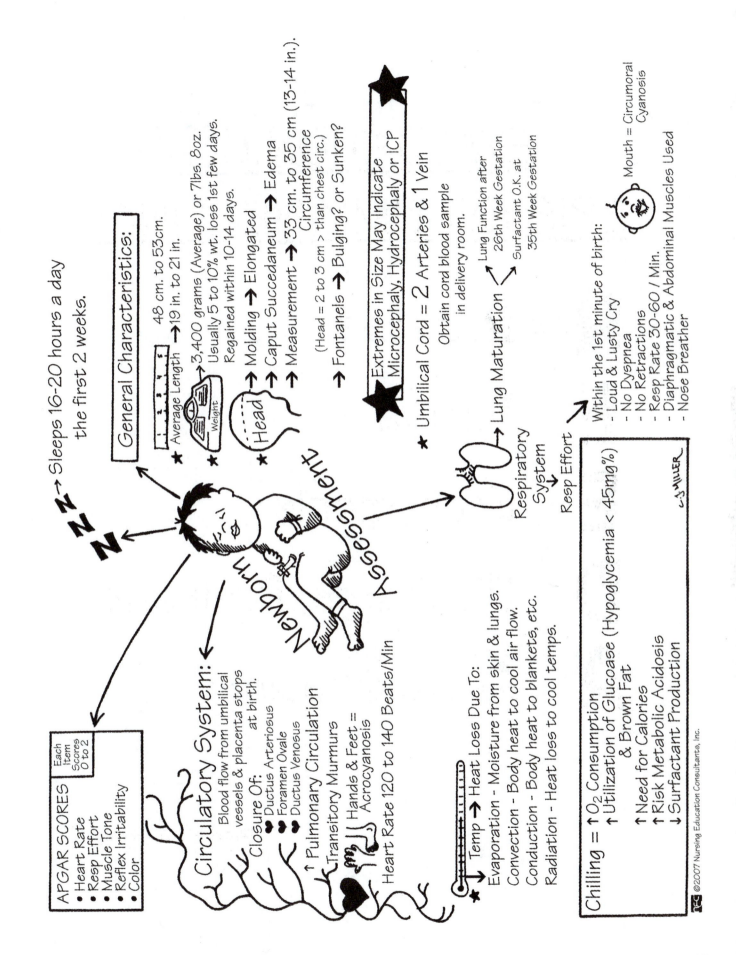

Newborn Assessment

→ Sleeps 16-20 hours a day the first 2 weeks.

General Characteristics:

★ Average Length → 48 cm. to 53cm.
→ 19 in. to 21 in.

★ Weight → 3,400 grams (Average) or 7lbs. 8oz.
Usually 5 to 10% wt. loss 1st few days.
Regained within 10-14 days.

★ Head
→ Molding → Elongated
→ Caput Succedaneum → Edema
→ Measurement → 33 cm. to 35 cm (13-14 in.).
Circumference
(Head = 2 to 3 cm > than chest circ.)
→ Fontanels → Bulging? or Sunken?

★ Extremes in Size May Indicate
Microcephaly, Hydrocephaly or ICP

★ Umbilical Cord = 2 Arteries & 1 Vein
Obtain cord blood sample
in delivery room.

Respiratory System

→ Lung Maturation
Lung Function after
26th Week Gestation
Surfactant O.K. at
35th Week Gestation

→ Resp Effort
Within the 1st minute of birth:
- Loud & Lusty Cry
- No Dyspnea
- No Retractions
- Resp Rate 30-60 / Min.
- Diaphragmatic & Abdominal Muscles Used
- Nose Breather

Mouth = Circumoral
Cyanosis

Circulatory System:

Blood flow from umbilical
vessels & placenta stops
at birth.

Closure Of:
- Ductus Arteriosus
- Foramen Ovale
- Ductus Venosus

↑ Pulmonary Circulation
Transitory Murmurs

Hands & Feet = Acrocyanosis

Heart Rate 120 to 140 Beats/Min

APGAR SCORES
| | Each Item Scores 0 to 2 |
- Heart Rate
- Resp Effort
- Muscle Tone
- Reflex Irritability
- Color

→ Temp → Heat Loss Due To:
Evaporation - Moisture from skin & lungs.
Convection - Body heat to cool air flow.
Conduction - Body heat to blankets, etc.
Radiation - Heat loss to cool temps.

Chilling = ↑ O$_2$ Consumption
↑ Utilization of Glucoase (Hypoglycemia < 45mg%)
& Brown Fat
↑ Need for Calories
↑ Risk Metabolic Acidosis
↓ Surfactant Production

C.J. MILLER

CEPHALHEMATOMA / CAPUT SUCCEDANEUM

Cephalhematoma:

Collection of blood between surface of a cranial bone and the periosteum membrane. <u>Does not cross suture lines.</u>

Caput Succedaneum:

C
R
O
S
S
E
S

S
U
T
U
R
E
S

Collection of fluid due to pressure of presenting part against cervix. <u>This crosses suture lines.</u>

From: Delores Graceffa, RN, MS

- HIGH RISK NEWBORN - NURSING INTERVENTIONS

TEMPERATURE

☆ Minimize Cold Stress.

☆ Maintain Skin Temp. 36.1° - 36.7°C (96.8° - 97.7°F)

☆ Continuously Monitor Temp.

☆ Prevent Rapid Warming or Cooling.

☆ Use A Cap To Prevent Heat Loss From Head.

RESP FUNCTION

☆ Position ↑O_2 - Semiprone/Side Lying

☆ Maintain Resp Tract Patency

☆ Stimulate → Remind to Breathe

☆ Monitor O_2 Therapy

☆ Assess Resp Effort
- Grunting
- Nasal Flaring
- Cyanosis
- Apnea

FOOD & FLUIDS

☆ Monitor For Hypoglycemia.

☆ Assess Tolerance Of Oral Or Tube Feedings.

☆ Monitor Hydration Closely.

☆ Assess For Gastric Residual, Bowel Sounds, Change In Stool Pattern, Abdominal Girth.

☆ Monitor Weight Gain Or Loss.

C.J. MILLER

TRACHEAL - ESOPHAGEAL FISTULA

(3C's)

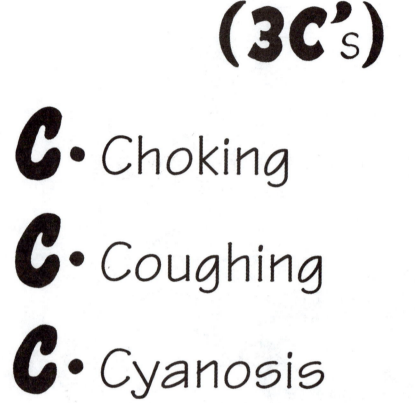

C. Choking

C. Coughing

C. Cyanosis

©2007 Nursing Education Consultants, Inc.

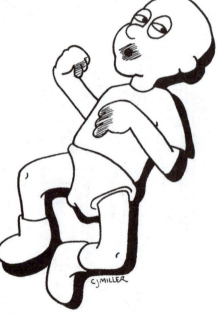

DEVELOPMENTAL DYSPLASIA OF THE HIP

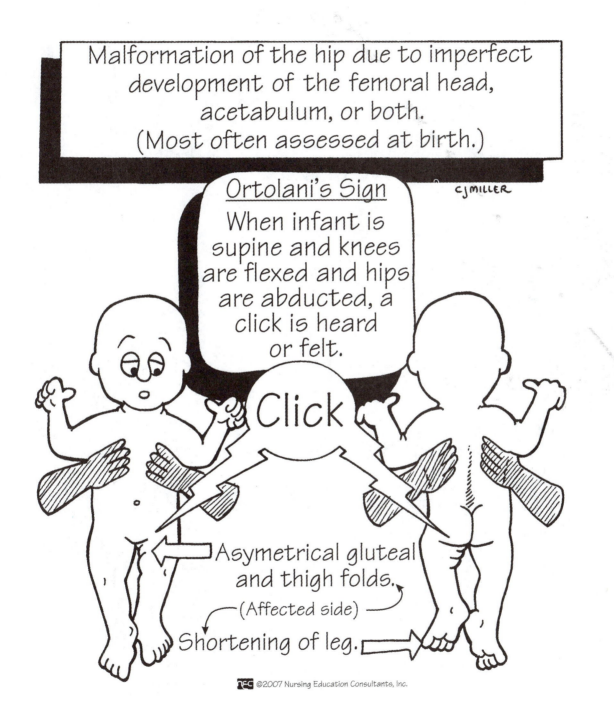

Malformation of the hip due to imperfect development of the femoral head, acetabulum, or both.
(Most often assessed at birth.)

Ortolani's Sign

When infant is supine and knees are flexed and hips are abducted, a click is heard or felt.

Click

Asymetrical gluteal and thigh folds.
(Affected side)
Shortening of leg.

131

CLEFT LIP - POST OP CARE

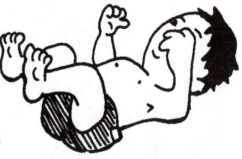

C Choking
L Lie on Back
E Evaluate Airway
F Feed Slowly
T Teaching

L Larger Nipple Opening
I Incidence ↑ Males
P Prevent Crust Formation

Prevent Aspiration

Antibiotic Ointment

IMMINENT DEADLINE STRESS DISORDER
(I.D.S.D.)

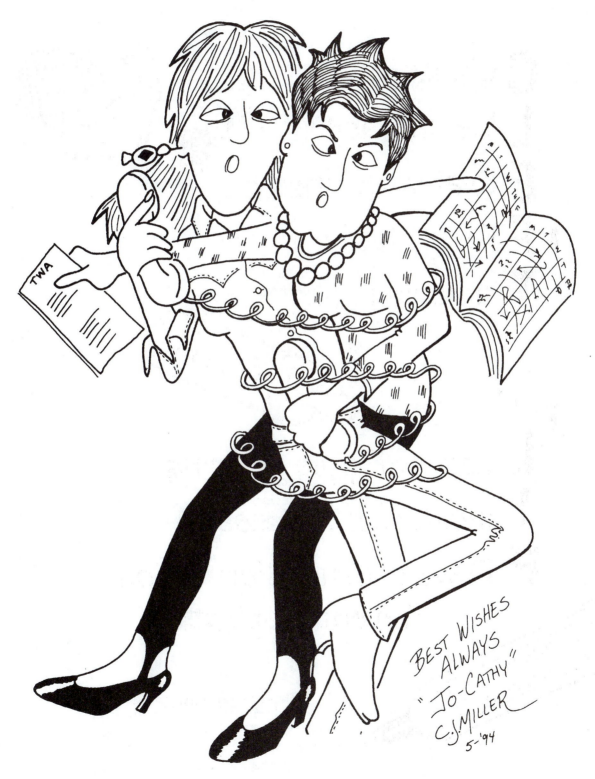

Index